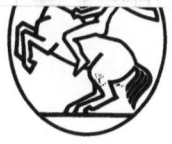

A. Harders

Neurosurgical Applications of Transcranial Doppler Sonography

Springer-Verlag Wien New York

Dr. med. habil. Albrecht Harders
Neurochirurgische Universitätsklinik Freiburg i. Br.,
Federal Republic of Germany

Product Liability: The publisher can give no guarantee for information about drug dosage and application thereof contained in this book. In every individual case the respective user must check its accuracy by consulting other pharmaceutical literature.

With 109 Figures

Library of Congress Cataloging-in-Publication Data. Harders, A. (Albrecht), 1947–   . Neurosurgical applications of transcranial Doppler sonography. Bibliography: p. Includes index. 1. Brain—Blood-vessels—Surgery. 2. Transcranial Doppler ultrasonography. I. Title. [DNLM: 1. Blood Flow Velocity. 2. Cerebrovascular Circulation. 3. Cerebrovascular Disorders—physiopathology. 4. Ultrasonic Diagnosis—methods. WL 355 H259n.] RD594.2.H37. 1986. 617′.481. 86-22007

ISBN-13: 978-3-211-81938-8   e-ISBN-13: 978-3-7091-8868-2
DOI: 10.1007/978-3-7091-8868-2

Foreword

In 1981, the Norwegian physiologist and cyberneticist, Rune Aaslid, developed a device which made it possible to apply the transcranial Doppler sonographic technique in man. In 1983, Dr. Albrecht Harders took on the project of working out a clinically practicable method that would allow atraumatic measurements to be made of the blood flow velocity in the large branches of the circle of Willis. The technique has now become a competitor of the conventional methods of measuring the intracranial hemodynamics, including angiography and the xenon method of cerebral blood flow measurement.

Harders proceeded from the assumption that the measurement of the blood flow velocity is more relevant for clinical diagnoses than the usual volume flow measurements. He stresses the very valuable application of the technique in detecting cerebral vasospasm before and after aneurysm surgery. The changes in the blood flow velocities measured by transcranial Doppler sonography in the individual vessel segments of the circle of Willis are interpreted with respect to the various factors that can effect such changes (collateral circulation in the circle of Willis, diameter of the vessel, vascular resistance, the general cardiovascular situation, arterial partial CO_2 pressure, autoregulatory factors, position of body). The rate of complications associated with angiography has thus been reduced, since the best time both for angiography and for surgery can be determined, and continuous TCD examinations show when the patient is out of a critical phase of cerebral vasospasm. The use of the TCD examination technique in Freiburg has significantly improved the postoperative course. Ischemic deficits are becoming more and more rare, as the indication for surgery and therapy (with hypertension) has become more defined.

The author has made an essential contribution to a very topical issue in neurovascular surgery.

Freiburg im Breisgau, July 1986   Wolfgang Seeger

Acknowledgements

I wish to express my sincere appreciation to my teacher, Professor Wolfgang Seeger, for having introduced me to the complex and limitless field of microanatomy and its applications in neurosurgery and thus making this study possible. I would also like to thank him for the excellent illustrations he has produced for this book.

Special thanks go to Dr. Rune Aaslid, who developed the prototype device for transcranial Doppler examinations and to Dr. Alec Eden for supplying us with the instrument with a minimum of red tape. The present study would have been impossible without the support of Dr. Aaslid (Bern, Seattle), Professor G.-M. von Reutern (Department of Clinical Neurology and Neurophysiology, Freiburg), and Professor J. M. Gilsbach (Department of Neurosurgery, Freiburg) whose support aided me in finding my way through the problems encountered in hemodynamics and Doppler sonography.

My further appreciation is extended to Professor Peter Huber of the Department of Neuroradiology in Bern, Switzerland, for allowing us to use his angiograph to determine vessel diameters; Professor J. J. Merland (Hôpital Lariboisière, Paris) made it possible for us to carry out transcranial velocity measurements during his excellent superselective AVM embolization procedures; Professor G. Meinig of the Department of Neurosurgery, University of Mainz (Head of Service: Professor K. Schürmann), who gave us the opportunity to perform CBF measurements and Doppler examinations on his patients with occlusive arterial disease.

I am further indebted to York Hilger for the setting up the computer program to present the numerous Doppler data. Finally, I should like to express my sincere thanks and admiration to Gerhard Pfister for his photography work which in some cases surpassed the quality of the originals; to Virginia Sonntag-O'Brien for the English translation; and to Inge Wurich and Hans Förster for their secretarial assistance.

Freiburg im Breisgau, July 1986   A. G. Harders

Contents

Introduction   1

Hemodynamic Principles   3
    Physiological Blood Flow   3

Principles of Ultrasound Doppler Sonography   6
    Doppler Formula   6
    Continuous Wave and Pulsed Doppler Instruments   6
    Insonation Angle   7
    Frequency Spectrum Analysis   8
    Vascular Resistance   9
    Ultrasound Doppler Sonography and Blood Flow Velocity   11

Transcranial Doppler Device   12
    Ultrasound and the Skull   12
    Technical Data   12

Transcranial Doppler Investigation Technique   16
    Anatomic Considerations   16
    Insonation Angle, Measured Depths, and Flow Direction   18
    Compression Tests   21

Normal Values   24

Blood Flow Velocity Changes Under Physiological Deviations   27
    Age   27
    Blood Flow Velocity End-tidal CO_2 Partial Pressure   28
    Orthostasis and TCD   29
    Body Acceleration   31
    Valsalva Test and TCD   31

*Spontaneous Subarachnoid Hemorrhage and Disturbed Intracranial
    Hemodynamics*   32
    Hemodynamic Considerations in Stenosis and Vasospasm   33
    Pathomorphology of the Cerebral Arteries After SAH and
        Vasospasm   33
    Timing of Aneurysm Operation   34

Natural Time Course of Vasospasm   35
    Patients   35
    Method   35
    Results   36

Vasospasm and Aneurysm Surgery Within 72 Hours After Subarachnoid Hemorrhage 40
  Introduction 40
  Patients 40
  Vasospasm Within 72 Hours After the Last SAH 42
  Vasospasm Between Day 4 and Day 31 After SAH 44
  Clinical Outcome 60
  Discussion 60

Correlation of Angiographically Confirmed Vasospasm and Stenosis with Transcranial Doppler 65

Vasospasm and Delayed Aneurysm Surgery 70

Intra-aneurysmal Flow Pattern 72
  Special Case: Vein of Galen—AVM 77

Extracranial-Intracranial Bypass 78
  Introduction 78
  Method 78
  Patients 79
  Results 80
  Results: STA Compression Tests and TCD 83
  Results: Special Cases 85
  Results: Comparison of CBF Measurements with Transcranial Doppler Sonography 87
  Discussion 88

Arteriovenous Malformations 94
  Introduction 94
  Feeding Arteries and Steal Effect 95
  SAH and AVM 98
  Vascular Resistance Following Surgical Exclusion 102
  Superselective Embolization and TCD Recordings 103
  Discussion 103

Monitoring of Frequency Spectra in the MCA During Angiography 108

Vascular Hemodynamic Response to Meningitis 111
  Introduction 111
  Case Reports 111
  Discussion 114

Brain Death and TCD Recordings 115

References 119

Subject Index 132

Introduction

The fact that ultrasound can penetrate the bony skull was utilized in the encephalographic technique. Nevertheless, for a long time the intracranial cerebral vessels could not be insonated using the conventional Doppler sonographic examination methods. In 1981, Aaslid developed a transcranial Doppler device with a pulsed sound emission of 2 MHz, which enabled blood flow velocities to be measured in the large branches of the circle of Willis. With this innovation it has become possible to record directly intracranial hemodynamic changes. Methods used until now to determine the intracranial hemodynamics include angiography, regional cerebral blood flow measurements with the [113]Xenon method, and the time-consuming positron emission tomography. Angiography remained the sole method of confirming cerebral vasospasm and subarachnoid hemorrhage after Ecker and Riemenschneider [52, 53] first reported their results of this application.

Until 1982, the Doppler sonographic technique was used only to measure the effects of intracranial vascular processes on the hemodynamics of the extracranial brain-supplying vessels [31,35]. Intraoperative Doppler sonography of the cerebral arteries was performed by Nornes, Moritake, Friedrich, and Gilsbach [65, 69, 138, 139, 147, 148, 150, 151, 154].

This book has been written to describe the various applications of transcranial Doppler sonography in neurosurgery. It describes the role of this still very young examination technique in the diagnostic and therapeutic procedures of cerebrovascular disease.

Hemodynamic Principles

Physiological Blood Flow

In rigid tubes with laminar flow and Newtonian fluids (the arterial system fulfills only the criterion for laminar flow), the following physical laws apply:

the Hagen-Poiseuille law

$$I = \frac{\Delta p \cdot r^4 \cdot \pi}{8 \cdot \eta \cdot L} \tag{1}$$

where I = the volume flow, which is measured in ml/min, Δp = the difference between the pressure at the beginning and at the end of the tube, r = the radius, π = the viscosity of the blood, η = a constant, and L = the length of the tube. The volume flow I = volume per time (t) and the volume is the product of the cross-section of the tube Q and the length.

$$I = \frac{\text{vol}}{t} = \frac{L \cdot Q}{t}. \tag{2}$$

The mean velocity of flow v in cm/sec is taken from volume flow and vessel radius:

$$v = \frac{I}{\pi \cdot r^2}. \tag{3}$$

The flow resistance R in a tube through which a fluid flows is dependent on the volume flow and the pressure gradient:

$$R = \frac{\Delta p}{I}. \tag{4}$$

If I is replaced with (1), the resistance is then

$$R = \frac{8 \cdot \eta \cdot L}{r^4 \cdot \pi}. \tag{5}$$

It is thus evident that even a small change in the diameter of the tube can cause a major change in the resistance.

These physical laws apply for rigid tubes with nonpulsatile flow of Newtonian fluids when there is no collateral flow. They are only partly applicable for pulsatile flow in the vascular system, which has numerous junctions, is controlled by autoregulation, and has a collateral capacity.

If (5) could be applied fully, the resistance in the arteries supplying the brain would thus increase with the 4th power of the radius, even when the diameter is reduced only slightly. This is prevented, however, by the autoregulation of the brain. The vascular resistance is adjusted by the arterioles and venules in such a way that at perfusion pressure gradients of between 60 and 150 mm Hg, there is constant cerebral flow [110, 111]. If the autoregulation becomes exhausted, equation (5) applies and a considerable increase in resistance with a reduction of flow then occurs, for example, in the case of a critical stenosis.

The diameter of the cerebral arteries ranges from 0.4 cm to 4 μm. The hemodynamics of the vascular system are determined by three physical properties: resistance, inertia, and compliance. These three properties have been summarized as impedance [189, 190].

1. *Resistance* (R) is caused by the loss of viscosity of blood as it flows through the vessels. Blood can only flow where a pressure gradient $\triangle P$ exists. The resistance is determined primarily in the small arteries and arterioles, or in the larger arteries if they are pathologically narrowed. The following equation applies:

$$R = \frac{128 \cdot \eta \cdot l}{\pi \cdot d^4}. \tag{6}$$

This means that very large vessels have very low resistance and vice versa. In the large vessels such as the internal carotid artery, resistance does not increase significantly until there is a lumen narrowing of at least 50%. The resistance is dependent to a large extent on the collateral circulation of a vessel. If the collateral circulation is poor, normal flow can be maintained up to a vessel diameter reduction of 2 mm. Further vessel narrowing causes a reduction of flow and can give rise to neurological deficits [188, 190].

If there is good collateral circulation in the presence of arterial stenosis, the blood flow decreases more rapidly at the site of the stenosis. The reason is that the pressure gradient does not rise, since the distal brain is supplied via the collaterals. If this pressure value is high enough to ensure normal perfusion, a vessel occlusion can occur without there being any symptoms of ischemia.

Besides the brain, another organ with low vascular resistance is the kidney. The arteries supplying the brain and the kidney therefore have a higher diastolic flow than the skin-supplying arteries.

2. *Inertia* appears mostly in large arteries and is caused by the mass of the blood. There is a delay between the increase in pressure and the resulting increase in velocity.

3. *Compliance* is a property of the arterial wall. It characterizes the ability of the arteries to expand during diastole and to accomodate a certain amount of blood volume. During systole, this blood is returned into the circulation. A typical example of compliance is the "Windkessel" function of the aorta.

Laminar flow in a vessel is characterized by the dimensionless Reynold's number (Re). Up to the critical value of 2,000 there is laminar flow. Beyond this value the flow becomes turbulent, for example, when there is low velocity of the blood, high density, wide vessels, or high flow velocity [48]:

$$\text{Re} = \frac{P \cdot D \cdot v}{\eta} \tag{7}$$

P = density of liquid
v = flow velocity
D = diameter of vessel
η = absolute viscosity

Prinicples of Ultrasound Doppler Sonography

In 1943, Christian Doppler published an article with the title "Über das farbige Licht der Doppelsterne und einiger anderer Gestirne des Himmels" [49]. The frequency of light and soundwaves is changed if the source and receiver are in motion relative to one another. The frequency increases when the source and receiver approach each other and decreases as they move apart. This physical principle became known as the Doppler effect. Details of the life and work of Doppler have been presented elsewhere by Eden [53].

Doppler Formula

Soundwaves undergo a change in frequency when the transmitter and the receiver move relative to one another. When the velocity of blood flow is measured, the ultrasonic waves are emitted from a transducer or probe and are backscattered by the red blood cells to be received again by the probe. The change in frequency, the so-called Doppler shift, is expressed by the following formula:

$$F = \frac{2 F_0 \cdot V \cdot \cos \alpha}{C} \tag{8}$$

where F_0 = determined frequency of the transmitted ultrasound, V = the real blood flow velocity, α = the angle between the transmitted sound beam and the direction of the blood flow, C = the velocity of sound in the tissue (1,550 m/sec in the soft tissue).

The blood flow velocity is proportional to the Doppler shift. The difference between the transmitted and reflected ultrasound is within the audible range and can be visualized with the aid of spectrum analysis.

Continuous Wave and Pulsed Doppler Instruments

With the so-called continuous wave (CW) instruments, the ultrasonic beam is continuously transmitted from one crystal and the backscatter is continuously received by another. This records frequency changes produced by all movements throughout the entire depth of penetration of the ultrasound. Inaccuracies can result when more than one vessel is insonated.

Ultrasound instruments with pulsed emission have now been developed that enable one vessel to be examined in isolation at a defined depth. One single crystal functions both as transmitter and receiver of the ultrasound wave. By means of the so-called electronic gate, the Doppler shifts are registered only at a certain distance from the probe and within a defined sample volume [17, 18]. When the sample volume is small, the vessel diameter can be judged with the aid of the electronic gate and the flow profile can be registered. This makes it possible to perform detailed measurements of the velocity distribution across the vessel diameter.

The penetration depth of the ultrasound in the tissue is inversely proportional to its frequency. To measure blood flow velocities at a depth of 7 cm from the surface of the skull, for instance, a low transmitting frequency of 2 MHz is suitable. When the frequency is low, however, the Doppler shift is also low, and the signal to noise ratio of the instrument is not favorable. The pulse repetition frequency (PRF) indicates at which time interval the sound pulse is transmitted from the crystal. The measuring depth and the maximum detectable Doppler frequency, which is half the PRF, are dependent on the PRF.

Insonation Angle

The angle at which the ultrasonic beam meets an intracranial vessel cannot be determined exactly. The Doppler shift measurements can be considered valid, however, since it can be safely assumed that the large arteries of the circle of Willis are insonated at an angle between 0° and 30°. The cosine value then fluctuates between 1 and 0.86, so that the error is less than 15% [1].

Fig. 1 shows the true velocity of the blood represented as a vector. The measured blood flow velocity is dependent on the angle between the ultrasonic beam and the axis of the vessel (formulas 1–4).

Thus, if the ultrasonic beam runs axially to the vessel, the true velocity of the blood is the same as the velocity vector. To be able to reproduce measurements in the Doppler sonographic examination on the vessels, an "optimum" vessel insonation angle always has to be obtained; in other words, the largest Doppler shift at the given depth.

If the Doppler examination is carried out intravasally, the ideal insonating angle, according to the Doppler formula, is 0°. If, however, a vessel is examined externally, the optimum angle is between 39 and 54° between the vessel lying parallel to the skin surface and the ultrasonic beam, as Kaneko reported in his experiments in 1970 [94]. This is due to the different reflections of the sound at the crystal, the red blood cells, and the vessel walls.

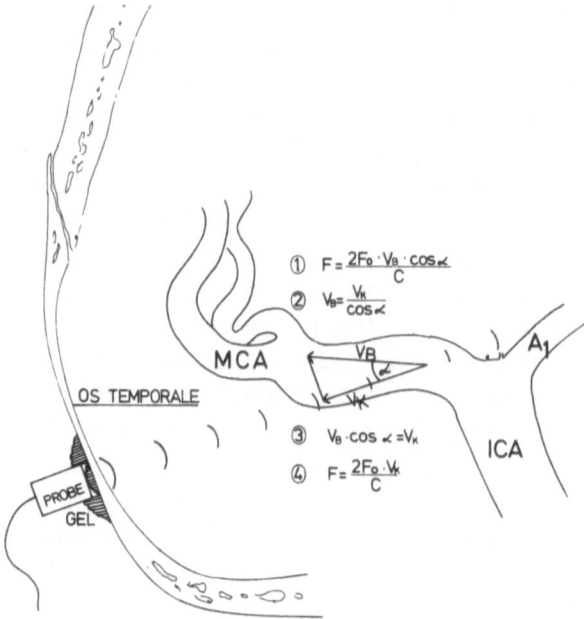

Fig. 1. Dependence of the Doppler shift (F) on the insonation angle of the middle cerebral artery. V_B true blood flow velocity, V_K velocity component

Because of this, Aaslid chose to express velocities in cm/sec, whereas in our studies we have retained the more traditional units of kHz Doppler shift, since it is this which is measured by the Doppler velocimeter. At an operating frequency of 2 MHz, the Doppler shift in Hertz can be converted to cm/sec by multiplying by 0.039.

The velocity of sound in the blood is dependent on the temperature, the protein content, and the hematocrit value. Within the measurable range of error, however, these dependencies can be disregarded and the velocity of sound in the blood under physiological conditions can be assumed to be about 1,565 m/sec [25].

Frequency Spectrum Analysis

The acoustic evaluation of the Doppler frequency spectrum provides information on turbulences and on changes in velocity and resistance.

The frequency spectrum can be represented in real time with the audiospectrum analysis [104, 127]. The advantage of this frequency analysis over the analogous mean frequency recording is that the maximum systolic and the minimum diastolic velocities, as well as the frequency distribution, can be represented in dependence on time. Orthograde and retrograde flow in the vessels can be simultaneously measured.

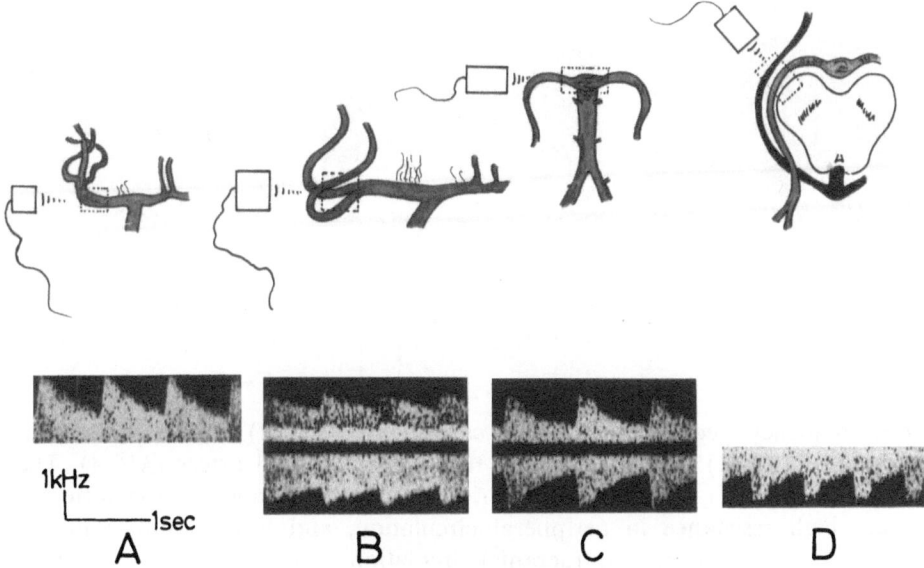

Fig. 2. Sample volume and measured velocities: *A* Frequency spectra of the proximal portion of the MCA-flow towards the probe. *B* Simultaneuous registration of velocities in three branches of the MCA. *C* Simultaneous registration of both precommunicating segments of the posterior cerebral artery. *D* Simultaneous registration of the postcommunicating segment of the posterior cerebral artery and the vena mesencephalica lateralis

With transcranial Doppler sonography, a sound emission of 2 MHz, and a sample volume larger than the recorded vessels, the frequency analysis registered all of the frequency ranges in a vessel section and a homogenous distribution of the frequencies in the spectrum is produced (Fig. 2).

Vascular Resistance

In 1960, Satomura and Kaneko [177] found differences in the pulse waveform during Doppler sonographic investigations of the common carotid artery and the facial artery. The arteries supplying the brain have a lower peripheral resistance than the external carotid arteries. That is why the cerebral arteries have a high diastolic flow velocity, whereas the external carotid artery has a low diastolic flow velocity. Pourcelot [160] characterized the flow pulse curve with the so-called "index of resistance" (R) (Fig. 3).

If in the recordings of the common carotid artery the R is greater than 0.75, an external type is indicated, which signifies a high peripheral flow resistance in the internal carotid artery. When there is an increase in the peripheral flow resistance and a reduction of perfusion pressure, as for instance in the case of increased intracranial pressure (edema, intracerebral

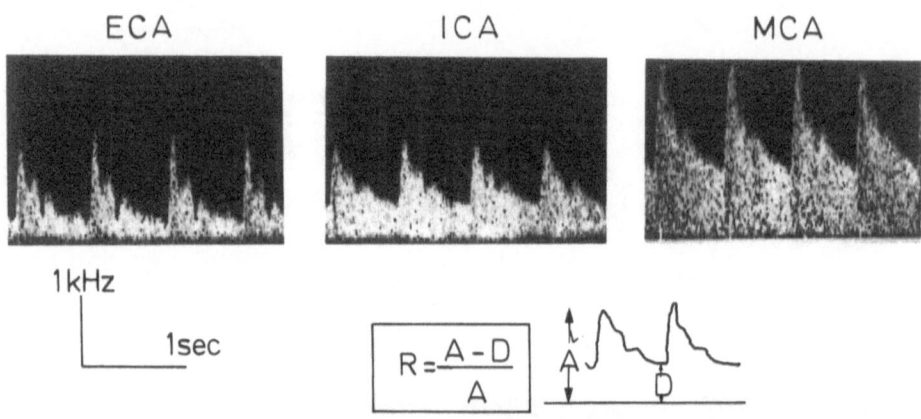

Fig. 3. Frequency spectra of the external carotid artery (*ECA*) in the neck, internal carotid artery (*ICA*) in the neck, and the middle cerebral artery (*MCA*). The resistance index (R) represents the varied vascular resistance in the different arteries, high resistance in peripheral circulation, and low resistance in the intracranial circulation

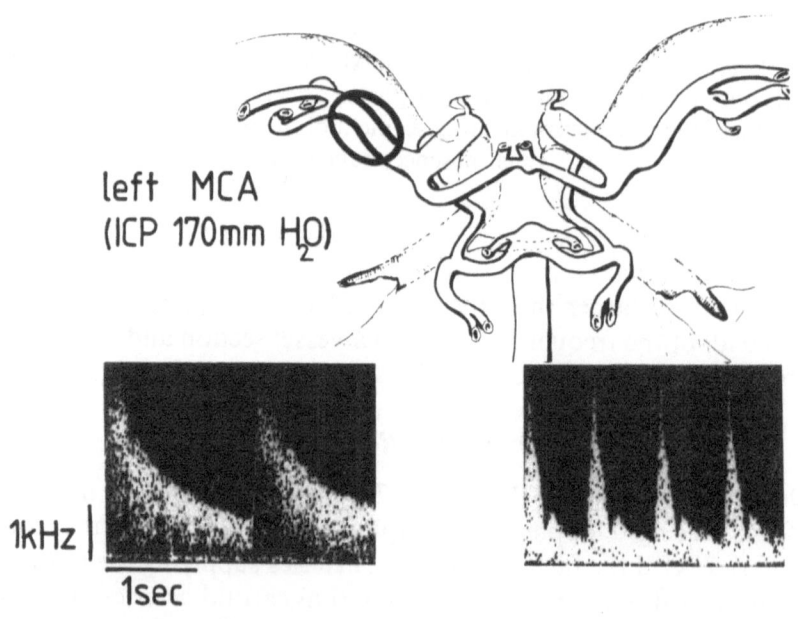

Fig. 4. Change in frequency spectrum before (left) and after (right) increased intracranial pressure has developed—high index of resistance due to hydrocephalus secondary to SAH

hemorrhage, hydrocephalus, Fig. 4), the flow pulse curve undergoes characteristic changes, from which diagnostic conclusions can be drawn. Greatly increased intracranial pressure occurs in brain death, in which the intracranial pressure corresponds to the systolic blood pressure.

Ultrasound Doppler Sonography and Blood Flow Velocity

In 1959, Satomura [176] used the Doppler method for the first time to investigate transcutaneously the velocities of blood flow in peripheral vessels. As early as 1960, Satomura and Kaneko [177] described the variation of vascular resistance. Mijazaki and Kato [137] also described the dependence of flow pulse curves on the peripheral resistance, functional tests on peripheral arteries, and changes in the flow pulse curves with increasing age. In the last 20 years, Doppler sonography has undergone rapid development in its application for the diagnosis of stenoses or occlusions of the extracranial cervical vessels and has become a standard procedure in clinical examination [10, 17–19, 22, 28, 30, 35, 57, 82, 92–95, 100, 115, 131, 149, 160, 163–170, 172, 190].

With extracranially applied Doppler sonography, only indirect hemodynamic effects of intracranial flow changes have been established. A reversal of the flow direction in the branches of the ophthalmic artery (supratrochlear artery and supraorbital artery) could be measured as a result of reduced perfusion pressure caused by stenosis or occlusion of the internal carotid artery [117, 131, 134, 138, 141–143].

Von Reutern [166] and Diener [45] investigated the increased flow velocities in the cervical arteries caused by intracranial angioma. Extracranial hemodynamic effects of fistulas of the cavernous sinus were described by Matejosko [132] and Büdingen [32]. Nornes [149], Büdingen [34], and Steiger [194] reported on the effects of raised intracranial pressure following head injury. Bradley [25] investigated the behavior of blood velocity under various physiological parameters and found that it is dependent, though only slightly, on temperature, total protein content, and hematocrit value.

Ultrasonic examinations of intracerebral vessels were carried out in children through the fontanelles and in adults through a trepanation hole [94, 140, 202]. Intraoperative Doppler investigations were performed during neurovascular operations by Brawley [27], Handa [77], Nornes [148, 150, 151, 155], Friedrich [65], and Moritake [139]. With the aid of a new microvascular pulsed Doppler instrument with a sound emission of 20 MHz, Gilsbach [69] obtained reliable values in vascular stenoses and occlusions during neurovascular operations.

Transcranial Doppler Device

Ultrasound and the Skull

In 1955, Leksell [116] found in making echoencephalographic recordings that ultrasound could penetrate the skull. Due to the reflection of ultrasound waves on the skull and on brain structures of various densities and sound conduction velocity, indirect space-occupying lesions could be demonstrated.

In 1965, Freund [64] registered the pulsation of the large branches of the circle of Willis using echoencephalography. In the presence of thrombosis of the internal carotid artery, a reduction of the vessel wall pulsation was recorded intracranially. It took until 1981, however, before the Doppler sonographic method could be used to measure the blood velocity in the brain vessels directly through the skull.

Technical Data

The Norwegian physiologist and cyberneticist, Rune Aaslid, developed a pulsed Doppler device with a transmitted frequency of 2 MHz, with which Doppler shift signals could be recorded through the skull. It could be empirically established that with a pulse group of 4–5 waves (burst-group) and a transmitted frequency of 2 MHz, the ultrasound waves were least scattered and sufficient reflecting sound energy could be registered.

The Department of Neurosurgery in Freiburg has been using a prototype of the transcranial Doppler device since 1983. The device has the following characteristics: pulse duration 16 ms, the same transmission and reception times, axial gate width (axial resolution) 10 mm at — 16 dB, gate width (lateral resolution) 4 mm at — 6 dB. The gate can be moved in steps of 5 mm from 2.5 to 7.5 cm from the probe. The pulse repetition frequency (PRF) remains constant at 7.88 kHz (Fig. 5).

Since the maximum Doppler shift frequencies detectable with the pulsed Doppler device are half the pulse repetition frequency, only blood flow velocities up to 4 kHz could be measured with the prototype device. Higher blood flow velocity caused an aliasing effect to occur [78, 79, 146, 171].

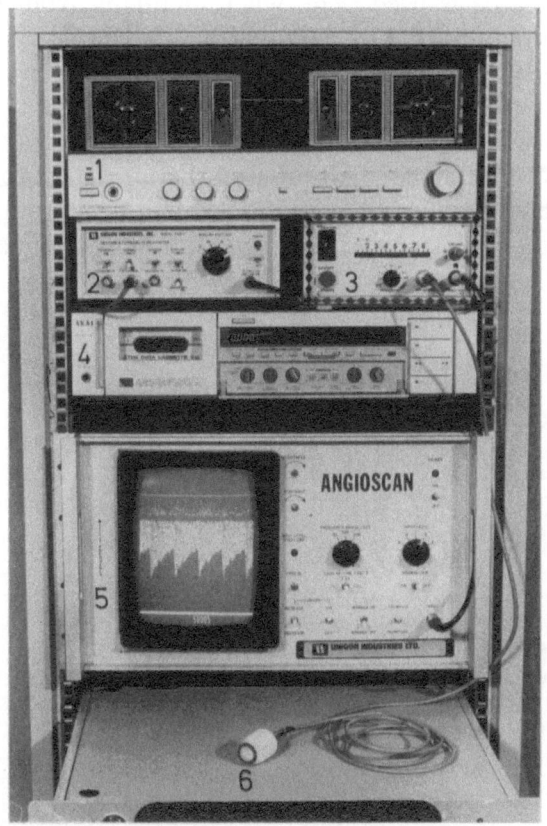

Fig. 5. Transcranial Doppler equipment: *1* Amplifier and loudspeakers. *2* Reverse and forward flow adapter. *3* Transcranial 2 MHz Doppler device (prototype). *4* Tape recorder. *5* Real time frequency analyzer. *6* Probe

With the later, commercially available TC 2–64 Transcranial Doppler (EME, Ueberlingen, West Germany), the pulse repetition frequency is electronically changed according to the measuring depth and scale setting, which allows frequencies up to 10 kHz to be obtained without aliasing (Fig. 6).

The monocrystal probe has a crystal diameter of 16 mm. The concave acoustic lens in front of the crystal serves to focus the beam of ultrasound at a nominal depth of 5 cm. The maximum transmitted sound energy is given as 100 mW/cm^2 by the manufacturer and can be adjusted in the following steps: 10, 25, 50, 75, and 100 mW/cm^2. The Bioeffects Committee of the American Institute of Ultrasound in Medicine recommends that the SPTA intensity (spatial peak, temporal average) should not exceed 100 mW/cm^2. This value will obviously be changed not only when the electrical power from the equipment to the probe is adjusted, but also when a probe with a different surface area is used (*e.g.*, when changing from transcranial to extracranial examination). For this reason, the intensity control switch controls the acoustic intensity as a percentage of the maximum output of the probe in use.

It is recommended that the least intensity necessary be applied to obtain an adequate Doppler signal. Although a better signal-to-noise ratio is usually achieved with higher intensities, a reduction will sometimes result in an improved signal with transcranial examination by eliminating overload-

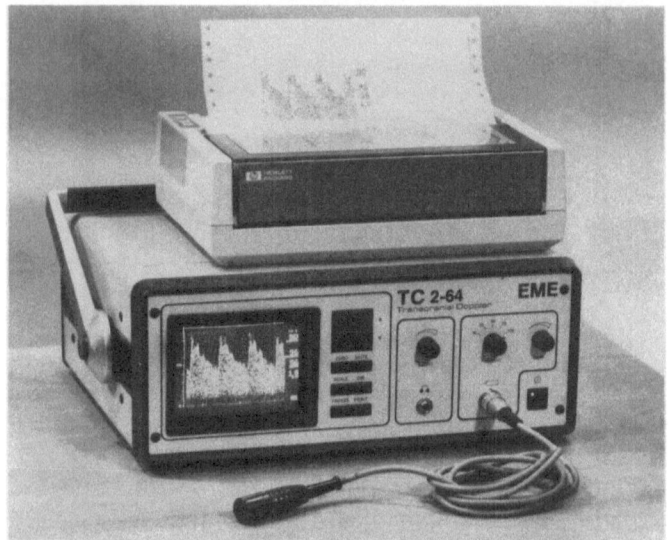

Fig. 6. The new transcranial Doppler 2 MHz device with built-in frequency analyzer and printer (EME, Ueberlingen, Federal Republic of Germany)

ing due to the reflection of ultrasound by the bony skull. Generally, SPTA intensities of between 50 and 100% are used for transcranial examination. For transorbital examination the intensity should not exceed 10%.

The evaluation of the Doppler signals was carried out with head phones or loudspeakers. With the prototype device, the Doppler frequency spectrum was analyzed with a real time frequency analyzer (Angio Scan I) and documented on Polaroid film. The TC 2–64 device has a built-in frequency analyzer and the spectrum can be printed out on a matrix dot printer. The equipment is bidirectional and in our investigations was set for the frequencies above the zero line to represent blood flow towards the probe.

The low transmitted frequency of 2 MHz makes it possible to measure flow velocities in intracranial basal cerebral vessels through thin "bony windows". With a maximum pulse repetition frequency of 20 kHz, velocities up to 10 kHz can be registered without aliasing. Doppler signals can be registered from a depth of between 2.5 cm to a maximum of 15 cm, thus enabling Doppler recordings to be obtained from both hemispheres during unilateral insonation.

Transcranial Doppler Investigation Technique

Anatomic Considerations

Usable Doppler signals can only be registered through thin "bony windows". By transillumination of the skull (Fig. 7), these windows can be demonstrated in the temporal bone, in the lateral part of the frontal bone, in the orbit, the orbital roof, and in the region of the suboccipital bone. Since the location and size of the cranial window varies with each person, the direction of the ultrasonic beam has to be adjusted individually in order to obtain optimum Doppler signals. The large basal arteries of the circle of Willis lie in a relatively narrow horizontal plane. Familiarity with the commonly occurring variations of the circle of Willis facilitates locating these vessels. Anatomic studies have revealed that only 53.8% of all persons have a "normal" circle of Willis [108]. The outer diameter and the length of each vessel segment are shown in Fig. 8.

"Normal" means: normal anterior communicating artery, normal posterior communicating artery, typical vessel branches, and a communicating artery no smaller than 1 mm in diameter. The most common variations include differences in diameter, course, and origin of the anterior and posterior communicating arteries. The direction of the middle cerebral artery is almost continuous with that of the internal carotid artery [109].

Pars praecommunicalis of the anterior cerebral artery (A1): hypoplasia of the A1 segment, diameter of 1 mm or less, appears in 8.6%, aplasia in 0.7–1.1%. Depending on the angle of origin from the internal carotid artery, the artery does not always run just horizontally (pars horizontalis of the mentioned A1), but can wind forwards, upwards, and downwards.

Anterior communicating artery: 74% of all persons have a classic anterior communicating artery. This vessel segment frequently has variations: 9% are doubled, 9% are Y-shaped, V-shaped, or plexiform. In the presence of a hypoplastic A 1, the postcommunicating segment is supplied by the widened contralateral A1 (general principle of cerebral dynamics). In only 0.3% is an anterior communicating artery absent.

Posterior communicating artery: if the lumen of the posterior communicating artery is larger than the precommunicating segment of the

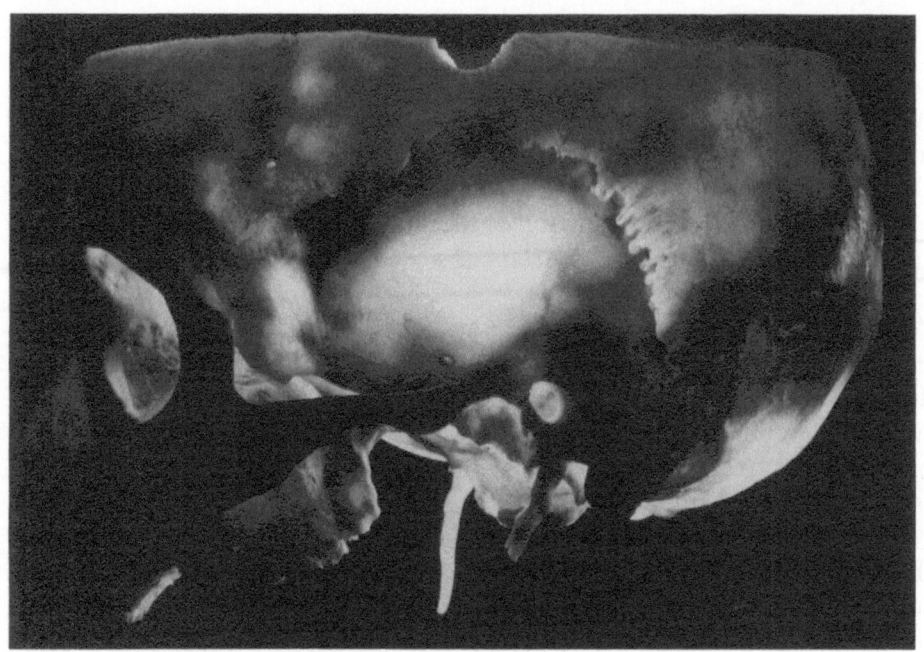

Fig. 7. Transillumination of the skull showing the "bony windows" in the temporal region and in the lateral part of the frontal bone

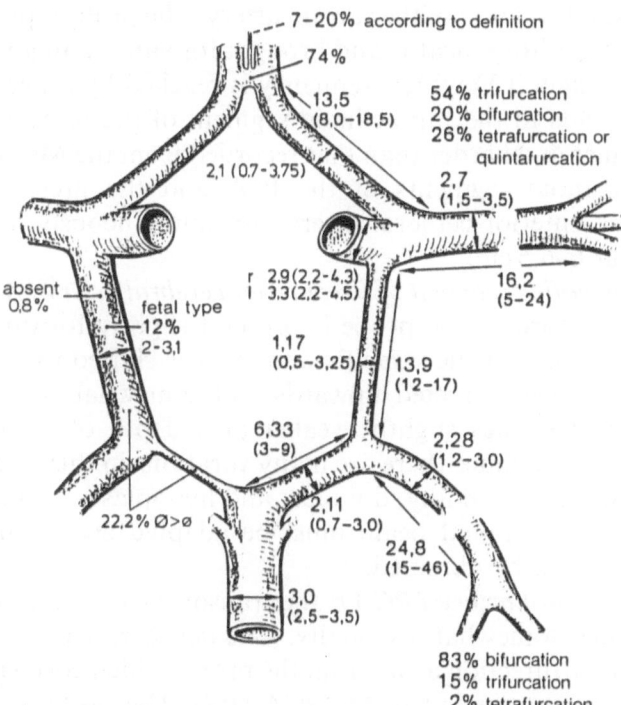

Fig. 8. Length and outer diameter of the cerebral arterial circle of Willis. (From Lang 1981 [108])

posterior cerebral artery, this is known as a fetal type (Lang: 12%). A direct junction of the posterior cerebral artery from the carotid artery can be anatomically proved in 10–35% [109]. Marked fluctuations in diameter of the posterior communicating artery and of the posterior cerebral artery can also occur in the posterior portion of the circle of Willis. According to Lang, the posterior communicating artery is absent in 1%.

Insonation Angle, Measured Depths, and Flow Direction

Middle cerebral artery (MCA): at the depth of 3–5 cm, reliable Doppler signals from the middle cerebral artery can be registered. Since the insular branches run at an obtuse angle to the ultrasonic beam, signals obtained from this vessel segment cannot be considered valid. The pars sphenoidalis of the MCA is insonated almost orthogradely from the sound beam when the probe is held behind the frontal process of the zygomatic bone and the sound beam is directed occipitally. The proximal portion of the MCA is usually reached through the bony window, which is located further back, approximately in the middle of the zygomatic bone. The sound beam must be directed upwards and slightly forwards.

Intradural segment of the internal carotid artery (ICA): after the proximal portion of the MCA is recorded at a depth of 4.5–5 cm, the pars supraclinoidalis of the ICA can be reached by means of range gating up to 6 cm above the bifurcation of the carotid artery. The probe is placed in front of the external auditory meatus and brought forward at an angle of about 30°. When the highest Doppler frequency is reached by range gating, this signal corresponds to the supraclinoid segment of the ICA. The sound is somewhat higher and harder than that recorded from the MCA. Frequently, the supraclinoid segments of the ICA and the precommunicating segment of the anterior cerebral artery are simultaneously recorded at a depth of about 6–6.5 cm.

Precommunicating segment of the anterior cerebral artery (A1): after the ICA has been recorded, the probe is brought slightly forward along the zygomatic arch while at the same time the gate is shifted to 6.5–7 cm. The beam then has to be directed upwards and somewhat posteriorly. The Doppler signal becomes slightly weaker at a depth of 6–7 cm and the direction is reversed. Since there are many varations in this vessel segment, such as ascending, descending, doubled, and hypoplastic forms of the A1, the direction of the sound beam must be adapted accordingly until an optimum signal can be obtained.

Posterior cerebral artery (PCA): the transducer is placed directly over the ear and tilted somewhat occipitally. At a depth of 5–6.5 cm, a signal is obtained with the direction away from the probe, which corresponds to the postcommunicating segment of the PCA (P 2). The probe is then slowly

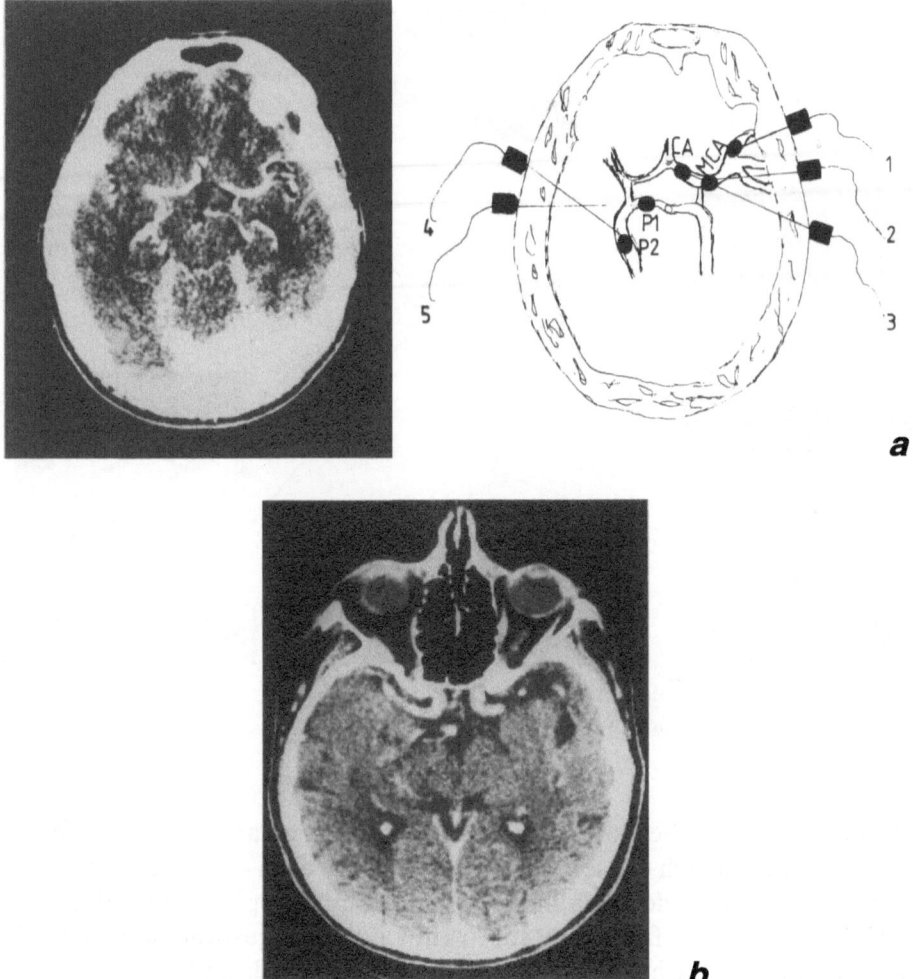

Figs. 9 a and b. *a* Cranial cerebral topography of the circle of Willis and the positioning of the probe to obtain an "optimal" insonation angle. *b* Cranial cerebral topography showing the supraclinoid segment of the internal carotid artery

brought forwards while the insonation angle is reduced until the direction of flow is towards the probe. The signal thus obtained stems from the homolateral PCA (P 1). When the gate is shifted deeper and the direction of flow changes, the contralateral P 1 segment is then being insonated. In most cases, low frequencies can be heard from the vein along with the pulsatile arterial frequencies, which correspond to the lateral mesencephalic vein (Rosenthal, Fig. 2 D).

Carotid siphon (transocular measurement): the emitted ultrasonic energy

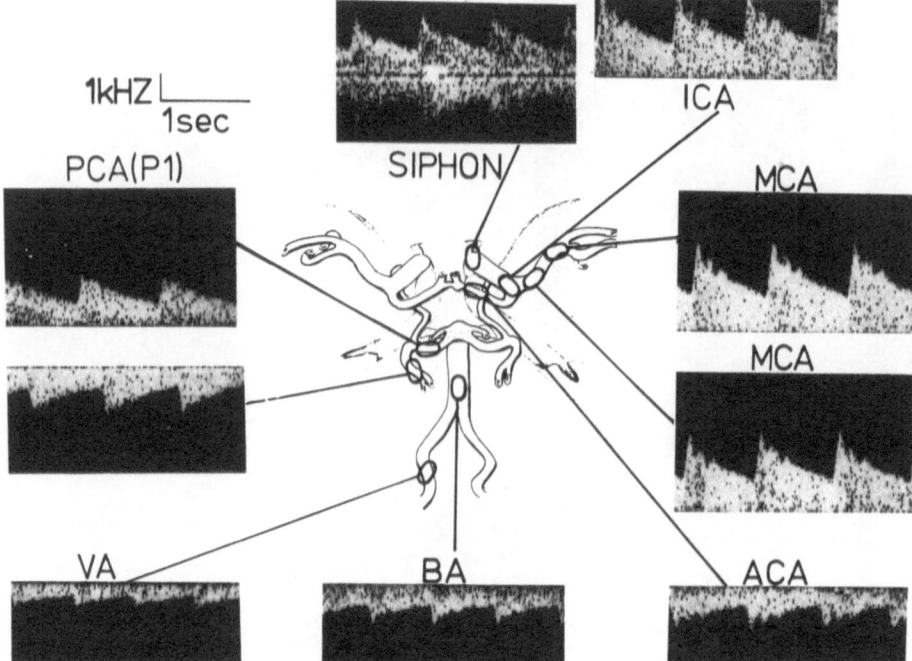

Fig. 10. Doppler frequency spectra from arteries of the circle of Willis with normal flow velocities and pulse waveforms

is reduced to 10%. The patient is instructed to look away from the probe so that the cornea, which causes scatter, is out of the path of the second beam. Examinations are made through the eyeball along the ophthalmic artery at a depth of 6–7 cm. The frequency spectrum with high diastolic flow depends on whether the probe is directed upwards or downwards and to the distal or the proximal segment of the carotid siphon. Flow towards the probe is more easily obtained (proximal segment of the siphon). By placing the probe in the lateral canthus and directing the beam towards the midline, one can record the homolateral segment of the A1 through the thin roof of the orbita [192].

A. vertebralis, intradural segment (VA): by placing the probe under the mastoid at a depth of 4–6 cm the intradural segment of the vertebral artery can be recorded. The Doppler signal indicates flow away from the probe.

A. basilaris (BA): the head is tilted forwards, the probe is placed in the midline between the occipital foramen magnum and arch of the atlas. When the sound beam is directed towards the bregma, it is lying in the direction of the basilar artery. This provides an almost orthograde insonation of the artery. In practice, however, an optimum Doppler signal is not achieved unless the probe is tipped somewhat caudally at a measuring depth of 8–

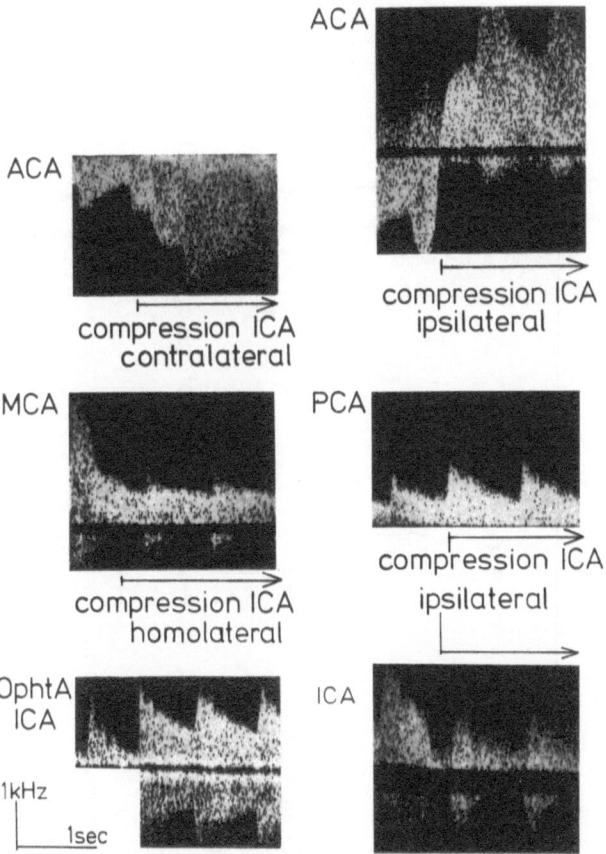

Fig. 11. Compression of the ipsilateral and contralateral internal carotid artery to identify the precommunicating segment of the anterior cerebral artery: flow velocity reduction in the middle cerebral artery, flow increase in the posterior cerebral artery, change in flow pattern from the ophthalmic artery to the carotid siphon, and reduction and reverse flow in the internal carotid artery

10 cm. Since the basilar artery often does not lie exactly in the midline, the probe is carefully tilted to the side to find the best Doppler signal.

In special cases (trepanation in the midline at the level of the bregma), the distal segment of the anterior cerebral artery (A 2) can be recorded through the trepanation hole, both at the level of the anterior knee of the corpus callosum (flow towards the probe) or further distally (flow away from the probe). Fig. 10 shows the frequency spectrum of normal cerebral arteries.

Compression Tests

The change in flow velocity and direction of the cerebral vessels during compression of the common carotid artery is an aid in identifying the vessel

Table 1. Identification of the recorded vessels with the help of depth, flow direction, and compression test. Orthograde: flow towards the probe; retrograde: flow away from the probe

Depth (cm)	Flow direction	Homolateral cervical ICA compression	Identified vessel
3–5	orthograde	reduction of Doppler shift	→ MCA
	retrograde	reduction of Doppler shift	→ ICA
5–6	orthograde	increase in Doppler shift	→ P1
	retrograde	no change in Doppler shift	→ P2
		reduction of Doppler shift	→ ICA
6–7	orthograde	increase in Doppler shift	→ P1
		reduction of Doppler shift	→ ICA
		no change in Doppler shift	→ A1 (occlusion of the opposite ICA?)
	retrograde	reversed flow	→ A1
		no change in Doppler shift	→ P2
		no change or increase	→ P1
7–8	orthograde	increase in Doppler shift	→ A1 contralat.
	retrograde	no Doppler shift	→ A1 (ICA occlusion homolateral?)
		no change in Doppler shift or increase in Doppler shift	→ P1 contralat.

and provides additional information on the collateral blood flow capacity of the circle of Willis (Fig. 11). The normal precautions that apply to compression tests should be observed.

MCA: the frequency spectrum of the MCA shows a greater or lesser reduction of the systolic and diastolic frequencies when the homolateral carotid artery is compressed. The pulse waveform is damped.

A1: when the anterior communicating artery is functioning adequately, compression of the ipsilateral common carotid artery will result in a reversed flow in the ipsilateral A1. Compressing the contralateral common carotid artery, on the other hand, results in a two-to threefold increase in the A1. No other artery in the circle of Willis shows this reaction at a depth of 7 cm.

ICA: when the ipsilateral common carotid artery is compressed, the flow ceases and retrograde flow of varying degrees appears.

P1: when the ipsilateral common carotid artery is compressed, the flow can increase as a result of a good collateral flow through the posterior communicating artery. If there is an embryonal type of posterior cerebral artery, the flow will cease.

The larger branches of the circle of Willis can be identified by the depth setting of the sample volume, the direction of the blood flow, the direction of the ultrasound beam, and by compression tests (Table 1).

Normal Values

Fifty persons with no clinical symptoms of cerebrovascular disease were examined. The ages of the patients ranged from 20 to 70 years. They were divided into five age groups (10 years each) with five women and five men in each. The patients were placed in a supine position with the head tilted forward about 30°. In three patients (6%), no usable Doppler signals could be registered through the skull. In the remaining cases, frequencies from the precommunicating segment of the ACA were recorded. Compression of the

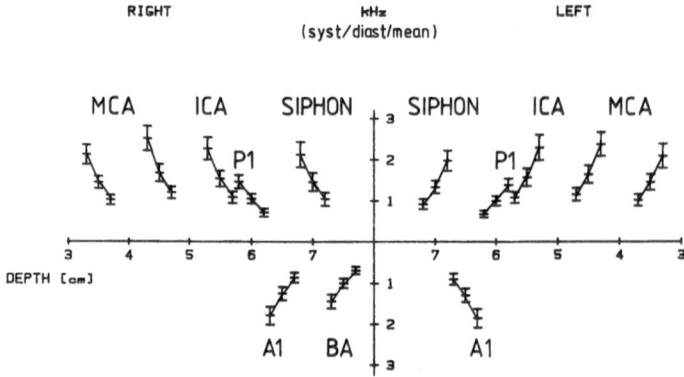

Fig. 12. Mean and standard deviation of the time averaged peak frequencies, peak frequencies, and diastolic frequencies of the different arteries of the circle of Willis in 50 healthy volunteers

contralateral common carotid artery resulted in a marked increase in the flow velocity (two- to threefold) indicating a well-functioning collateral system via the anterior communicating artery.

Table 2 shows the mean values (M) and the standard deviations (SD) in the individual segments of the circle of Willis measured in kHz. Systolic, diastolic, and time-averaged peak frequencies.

The schematic representations in Fig. 12 illustrate the almost identical velocity distribution in the two hemispheres. The minimal standard deviation is an indication of the reliability of the investigation method. The highest flow velocities are present in the proximal segments of the MCA and

Table 2. Normal transcranial Doppler shifts in 50 persons: mean (M) and standard deviation (SD) from the recorded parts in the circle of Willis

Vessel	Depth (cm)	Systolic		Mean		Diastolic		Side
		M	SD(±)	M	SD(±)	M	SD(±)	
MCA	3.5	2.12	0.48	1.45	0.30	1.02	0.24	R
		2.08	0.59	1.45	0.39	1.01	0.28	L
MCA	4.5	2.52	0.60	1.68	0.43	1.20	0.29	R
		2.37	0.58	1.64	0.43	1.15	0.32	L
ICA	5.5	2.27	0.55	1.54	0.39	1.08	0.28	R
		2.29	0.62	1.57	0.43	1.08	0.27	L
Siphon	7.0	2.12	0.62	1.46	0.44	1.04	0.32	R
		1.98	0.49	1.34	0.31	0.92	0.25	L
PCA (P1)	6.0	1.46	0.32	1.05	0.24	0.71	0.20	R
		1.39	0.31	1.00	0.23	0.68	0.18	L
ACA (A1)	6.5	1.79	0.45	1.25	0.32	0.86	0.24	R
		1.86	0.47	1.29	0.33	0.90	0.27	L
BA	7.5	1.44	0.34	1.00	0.23	0.69	0.18	

R = right side, L = left side

in the distal ICA, the lowest velocities are in the basilar artery and in the A 1 and P 1 segments. There are no differences in the Doppler frequencies based on sex and the side of the brain recorded.

Taking into consideration the cranio-cerebral topography of the possible variations in the circle of Willis, satisfactory Doppler signals from the individual segments of the circle of Willis can be recorded in about 94%. It might be possible in the future to obtain a higher percentage of positive recordings by selecting an emission frequency of 1.5 MHz. Our results correlate with the normal values published by Aaslid in 1982 [1] and the findings of Arnolds and von Reutern [9]. By measuring the highest Doppler frequency at a prescribed depth, comparable values can be reproduced. During direct intraoperative measurements, Gilsbach [69] was also able to show that the highest Doppler frequencies can be found in the proximal MCA and in the supraclinoid portion of the ICA.

Blood Flow Velocity Changes
Under Physiological Deviations

Age

In 50 persons with no clinical signs of vascular disease, the blood flow velocities in the basal arteries were measured to examine the connection between flow velocity and age (Fig. 13). The results of the measurements

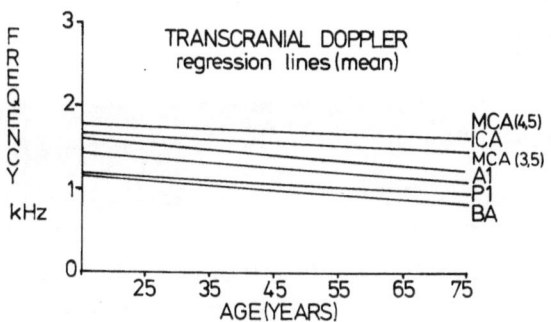

Fig. 13. Regression lines showing the relation of flow velocities to age in the different arteries. There is a statistically significant reduction of the flow velocity in MCA (3, 5), A1, P 1, and basilar artery

showed that the flow velocities were higher among the group of volunteers betweeen 20—30 years of age than in the group of persons between 60 and 70 years of age: in the MCA (3.5) there was a 20% reduction, in the MCA (4.5) 10%, in the ICA 10%, in the A1 20%, in the P1 15%, and in the basilar artery 25%.

Using the quantitative blood flow measuring system (QFM), [68] Fuhishiro [66] found that with increasing age the common carotid artery becomes wider and the flow velocity in this vessel and the flow volume are reduced. Cerebral flow measurements [136] have shown that a marked reduction of flow takes place with age. Thus, both the reduced brain perfusion and the increase in the vessel caliber are responsible for the reduced blood flow velocities measured transcranially in the circle of Willis in older persons.

Blood Flow Velocity End-tidal CO₂ Partial Pressure

Changes in the arterial CO_2 partial pressure have a substantial effect of the blood flow in the brain, as Reivich [162], Sokoloff [186] and Lassen [112] have shown. Huber *et al.* [85] studied changes in the diameter of the cerebral vessels during hypoventilation and hyperventilation on the basis of

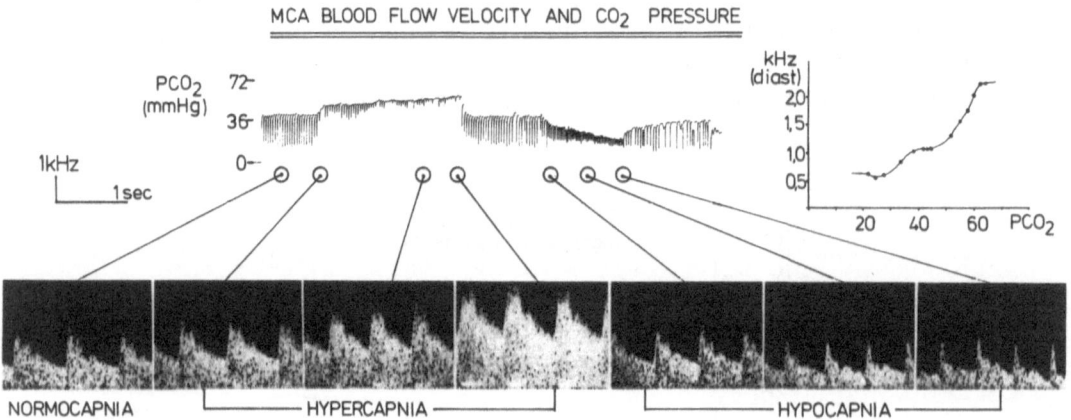

Fig. 14. Reaction of flow velocity in the MCA to end-tidal carbon dioxide partial pressure (PCO_2) in a 38-year-old man

angiographic findings. The vessels with a diameter of 0.5 to 1 mm reacted to pCO_2 changes by becoming wider, while basal arteries larger than 2.5 mm in diameter showed no such reaction.

Using transcranial Doppler sonography, Markwalder [130] was the first to describe changes in blood flow velocities in the MCA induced by end-expiratory pCO_2 changes.

Figs. 14 and 15 provide examples of the changes in the frequency spectra brought about by hypocapnia and hypercapnia. Hypocapnia can reduce the diastolic velocity to 0.5 kHz or can even result in zero flow in early diastole. In the presence of hypercapnia, the diastolic velocity rises to 2—2.5 kHz.

The changes in flow velocity caused by CO_2 reactivity of the vessels must be taken into account when interpreting the transcranial Doppler findings, particulary in the case of intubated and mechanically ventilated patients.

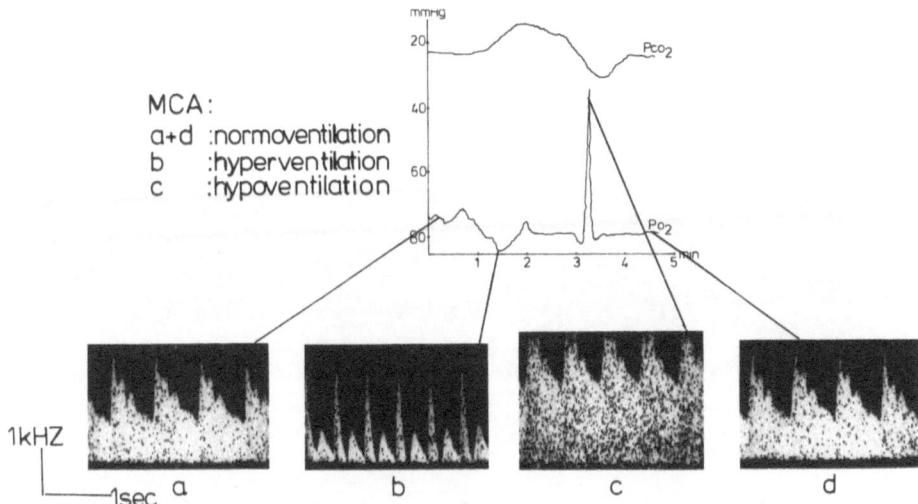

Fig. 15. Change in flow pattern in the MCA in a 28-year-old woman during hypocapnia (*b*) and hypercapnia (*c*). During hypocapnia there is early diastolic zero flow (*b*) and during hypercapnia an increase in diastolic flow up to 2 kHz (*c*). The PCO_2 and the PO_2 were measured transcutaneously (Radiometer Kopenhagen TCM/20/200). The PCO_2 does not show the correct absolute value but illustrates the relative changes

Since the diameter of the large cerebral arteries is not influenced by hypercapnia and the blood pressure rises only slightly, blood flow velocity measurements are able to provide conclusive information on changes in flow volume. In the presence of arteriovenous shunts (arteriovenous malformations, arteriovenous fistulas), there is no or only limited vascular reactivity to CO_2. This factor can be used as a criterion for diagnosing such diseases.

Orthostasis and TCD

When a person suddenly changes position (*e.g.*, from sitting to standing), the velocity of blood flow temporarily increases in systole and decreases in diastole. This observation is based on measurements made on the common carotid artery [35].

Continuous registration of the blood flow velocity in the MCA (Fig. 16) shows that the diastolic flow velocity is considerably reduced for approximately 3 seconds when a person stands up abruptly. Afterwards there is a progressive increase in both the diastolic and the systolic velocities as a result of reactive hyperemia. After 10–12 seconds the frequency spectrum returns to normal.

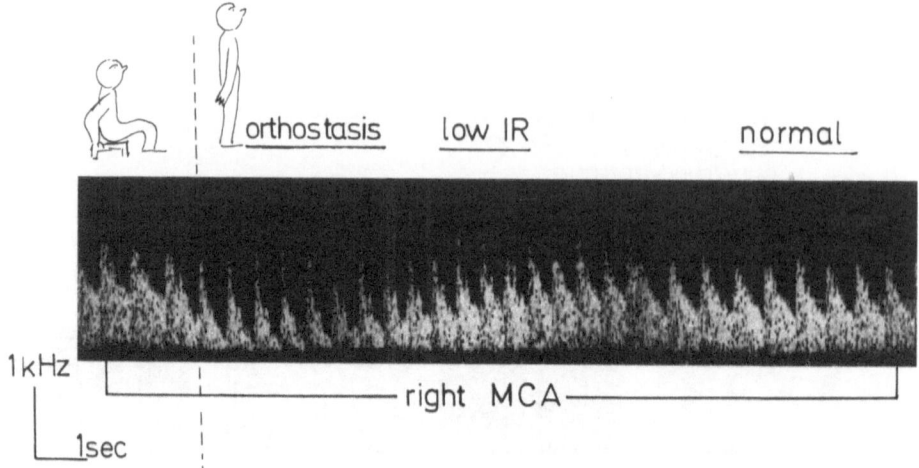

Fig. 16. When the person lying or sitting changes quickly to an upright position the diastolic flow velocity and the blood pressure decrease considerably as a result of orthostasis. As hyperemia occurs, the blood flow velocity increases and the flow pattern returns to normal within 11 seconds

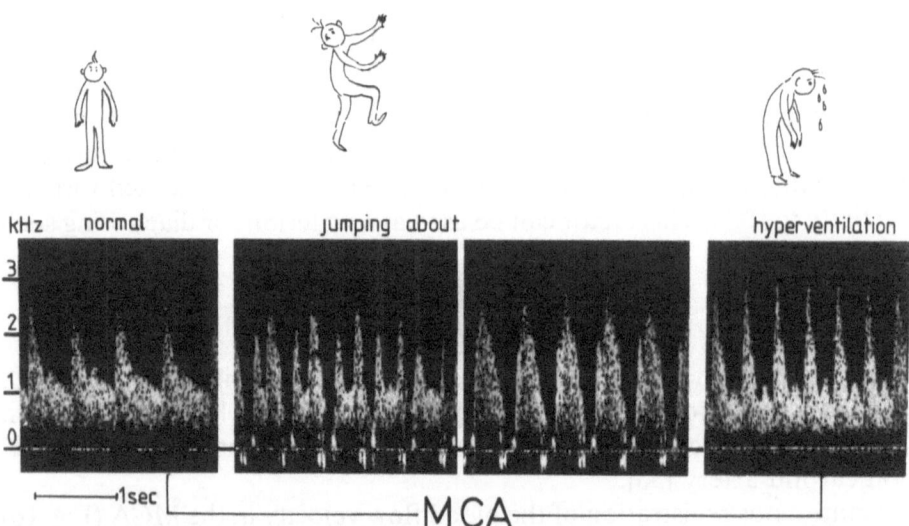

Fig. 17. Artificial change in the flow pattern in the MCA while jumping about: depending on the height of the jumps, single—or double—peaked systolic velocities may appear, the diastolic flow is zero for a short time, and there are no signs of reverse flow. When the jumping is stopped, increased vascular resistance due to hyperventilation can be observed

Body Acceleration

During body acceleration (*e.g.*, hopping and jumping), the frequency spectra show various velocity profiles, depending on the degree of acceleration. Fast hopping usually brings about a brief diastolic zero flow (Fig. 17). Depending on the time course of the acceleration, single-, double-, or multi-peaked systolic velocities can be registered. The low frequencies recorded above and below the zero line and which appear white are artefacts that were caused when the Doppler probe was moved during the acceleration.

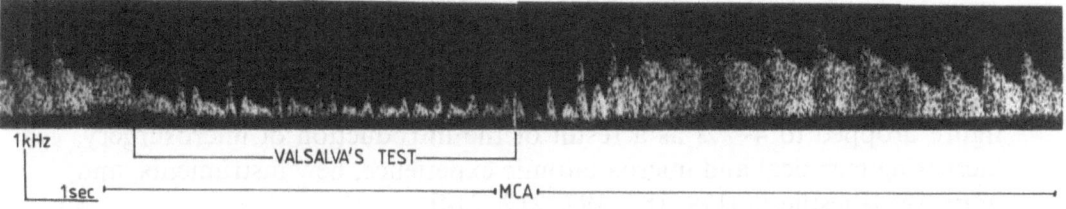

Fig. 18. Valsalva test and blood flow velocity in the MCA. During the tests, the blood flow velocity decreases considerably as a result of increased intracranial pressure due to restricted backflow of venous blood. Afterwards there is an increase in flow velocity due to hyperemia and the the flow pattern returns to normal.

Valsalva Test and TCD

During the Valsalva test (Fig. 18), reduction of both systolic and diastolic velocities is observed as a sign of increased intracranial pressure. After the test has been completed, diastolic and systolic velocities increase to just above normal, denoting brief reactive hyperemia.

Spontaneous Subarachnoid Hemorrhage and Disturbed Intracranial Hemodynamics

When the surgical clipping of cerebral aneurysms was in its infancy, the operation mortality was 50%, which was no better than the mortality rate of those patients who did not undergo acute aneurysm surgery [123]. This figure dropped to 4–7% as a result of the introduction of microsurgery, increasing technical and microanatomic experience, new instruments, and improved anesthesia [179–183, 197, 212, 214].

Apart from postoperative bleeding, cerebral vasospasm is the major cause of morbidity following subarachnoid hemorrhage in 10–30% [97, 121, 123]. While the clinical picture following SAH has been adequately studied, the actual pathomechanism of vasospasm is still unclear, despite extensive experimental investigations [5–7, 24, 26, 61, 67, 74, 84, 98, 102, 119, 175, 206, 210]. What is certain, however, is that vasospasm is caused by the blood in the subarachnoid space and its decomposition products.

Until now, vasospasm could only be diagnosed by angiography [51, 52]. For patients with vasospasm, however, angiography is about 5–10 times more dangerous than for those without [50, 86, 129, 158]. Extensive angiographic investigations [103, 173, 205] established the incidence distribution. In the first three days there is hardly any occurrence of vasospasm, after which the incidence increases up to the 9th to 12th day, reaching a maximum between day 10 and day 17, and then subsiding up to day 41.

Apart from angiography and clinical diagnostic methods, only very complex and time-consuming procedures are available to detect the consecutive symptoms of vasospasm, such as computed tomography, regional cerebral blood flow measurements, the ^{133}Xenon method, or positron emission tomography. In 1983, Meyer [136] observed in daily cerebral blood flow measurements a continuous reduction of flow in the first 14 days after SAH, after which there was a slow increase. Transcranial Doppler sonography makes it possible for the first time to selectively measure the hemodynamic effect of vasospasm, namely, the increased blood flow velocity.

Hemodynamic Considerations in Stenosis and Vasospasm

According to the law of continuity, in a vessel with no or only minimal collateralization which has become stenosed, the inflowing volume per time is identical to the outflowing volume per time. Thus the continuity equation applies:

$$Q1 \times V1 = Q2 \times V2$$

where Q = the diameter of the vessel, V = the flow velocity. The type of stenosis causes either a laminar or turbulent flow [188–190]. If the vessel becomes dilated directly beyond the site of stenosis, a drop in pressure occurs with turbulence and retrograde flow at the vessel wall. Severe stenoses that extend over just a short distance can also result in turbulences and poststenotic vessel wall vibrations. In the case of moderate stenoses over a longer distance, the laminar flow can be maintained. Spencer [189] investigated the theoretical relationship between the velocity and the volume of flow various degrees of stenoses, based on the cervical ICA. He discovered that a substantial reduction of the flow volume does not take place until there is an 80% lumen reduction (so-called critical stenosis). The increase in flow velocity caused by the stenosis, however, occurs much sooner. From the critical degree of stenosis on, the flow velocity decreases rapidly.

The critical degree of the stenosis is greatly influenced by the collateral circulation. The lower the resistance in the collateral circulation, the lower the flow velocity in the stenosis. The continuity equation can be applied when the autoregulation is intact and when there are few collaterals, as in the MCA, for example. In other words, when the lumen of the vessel is reduced by half, the flow velocity is doubled. In measuring a vessel with good collateralization, *e.g.,* the precommunicating segment of the ACA or the PCA, this equation can only be used conditionally. The complex relationships between blood flow velocity and collateral flow in the presence of intracerebral stenoses or occlusions must be taken into account when interpreting the Doppler sonographic measurements of intracerebral flow velocity.

Pathomorphology of the Cerebral Arteries After SAH and Vasospasm

According to autopsy findings in man [41, 87, 184, 185], in the first three weeks after subarachnoid hemorrhage there is edema of the tunica adventitia, necroses in the tunica media, irregularities in the tunica elastica, and swelling of the tunica intima. Late vessel wall changes after the 26th day after SAH include considerable wall thickening with increased connective tissue in the tunica adventitia, atrophy of the tunica media with slight fibrosis, thinning and irregularities of the tunica elastica. Most damage is done to the subendothelial fibrosis of the tunica intima with a thickening of the vessel wall, so that primarily the outer diameter of the vessel is enlarged. On the basis of histological findings, it is assumed that after subarchnoid hemorrhage, a vasospasm causes constriction of the vessel wall thereby inducing hypoxic changes in the vessel wall with thickening.

Animal experiments [23, 40, 54, 55, 96] have shown that the following pathomechanisms are triggered off after subarachnoid hemorrhage and vasospasm:

1. initial muscle contraction of the arterial wall,
2. endothelial desquamation with thrombocyte adhesions,
3. repair process with proliferative arteriopathy and thickening of the vessel wall.

Apart from morphological narrowing of the cerebral arteries after SAH, the following pathophysiological events can occur, all of which have an effect on the cerebral circulation: Increased intracranial pressure due to disturbed circulation of the CSF [105], cerebral edema, reduced cerebral blood flow, increase in the intracranial blood volume, and hypertension [16].

Timing of Aneurysm Operation

In order to prevent repeated aneurysm rupture and to guarantee adequate treatment of vascular spasm in the second week following subarachnoid hemorrhage, it is becoming more and more common to clip the aneurysm within the first 72 hours after SAH [11, 12, 121, 122, 174, 197, 198, 201]. In our department, we have been performing early surgery for aneurysms since 1979.

Natural Time Course of Vasospasm

Angiographic investigations [103, 173] have provided the following information on the incidence of vasospasm: in the first three days after subarachnoid hemorrhage, vasospasm occurs in 0–4.2%, after which the incidence increases up to the 7th and 10th day, the maximum is reached between the 11th and 17th day. After this, the occurrence of vasospasm falls. These results were obtained in patients who had undergone angiography only twice or, at the most, three times, as angiography poses a high risk for patients with vasospasm [50, 86, 128, 129, 158].

Up to now there has been no objective investigation technique to follow the time course of vasospasm. Recording the flow velocities in the circle of Willis using the transcranial Doppler sonographic technique is a sensitive method of measuring the effect of vasospasm, namely, the increase in velocity. The individual time course of vasospasm can now be traced.

Since we treat aneurysms by early surgery (= operation within 72 hours after SAH), we only have measurement data from a limited number of patients.

Patients

Twelve patients with subarachnoid hemorrhage were controlled by transcranial Doppler investigation without surgery. In six cases, angiography did not reveal an aneurysm. Angiography was postponed in five cases on the basis of the Doppler findings (time averaged peak frequencies above 3 kHz). In one case, surgery was put off because an aneurysm had already been determined. The severity of the SAH in CT was divided into three stages (modified according to Fischer [59].

Method

Transcranial Doppler recordings were performed at short intervals (at least every three days). Frequencies were measured in the MCA, in the supraclinoid portion of the ICA, in the carotid siphon (transorbital approach), in the proximal segment of the anterior cerebral artery (A1), and in the precommunicating segment of the posterior cerebral artery (P 1). The time averaged peak frequencies were used for further evaluation of the Doppler signal.

The statistical method selected for calculating a representative curve showing the time course of the velocity changes was the "spline approximate" procedure. The times were replaced by their arithmetic mean values and the standard deviation for each mean value was calculated. The curve was calculated in such a way that the points of higher reliability were approximated more closely and the points of lower reliability less closely. As a measure for the reliability of a point, the standard error of the daily mean

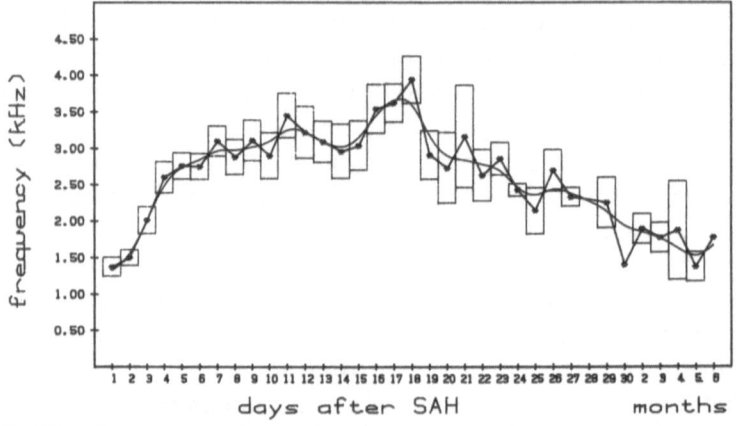

Fig. 19. The day mean values of 29 patients suffering severe SAH (CT = 3) are directly corrected. The calculation of a smooth curve as close as possible to the values and the standart error at the different days are presented

value was used. Each measured value (day mean value) thus received a weight, which was inversely proportional to the standard error, so that the points of higher reliability were given greater weight and the points of lower reliability a lower weight. Finally, a "smoothing spline function" based on local cubic polynomials was calculated in such a way that the integral of the error squared was minimal (Fig. 19). CT grading of the SAH, which was modified according to Fischer [59], is represented in Table 3.

Results

The measurements of the frequency changes in the first four weeks after SAH shows that these changes are most pronounced in the MCA and in the supraclinoid portion of the ICA (Figs. 20 and 21). The least changes were found in the posterior cerebral artery. The frequency increase started between the 4th and 12th day after SAH, the peak was reached between the 13th and 20th day, after which the frequencies slowly returned to normal. The changes in the frequency spectra are shown in Fig. 22.

Table 3. Grading of the severity of SAH in preoperative CT

Grade	Extent of SAH on preoperative CT
I	thin localized layer
II	thick layer in 2 of the 3 subarachnoidal compartments (basal cisterns, Sylvian fissures, interhemispheric space) or 1 subarachnoidal compartment and cortical surface
III	severe diffuse SAH with thick layer in all 3 subarachnoidal compartments or 2 and cortical surface

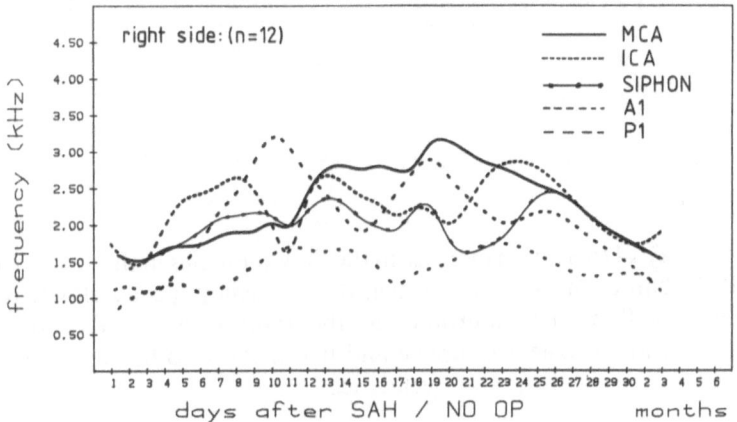

Fig. 20. Natural time course of frequency changes in the different arteries on the right side following SAH without surgery

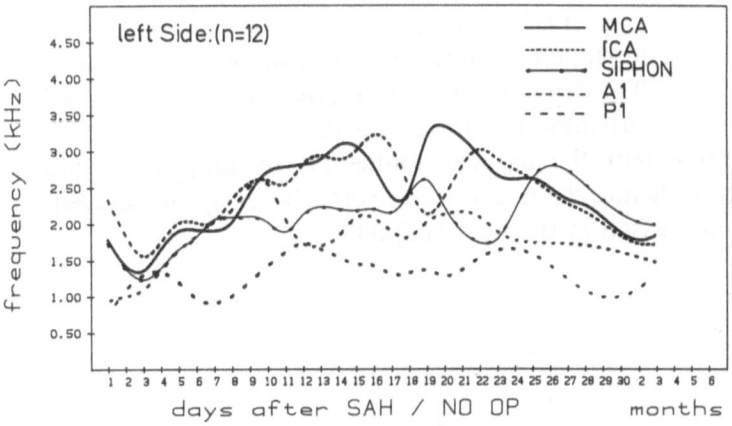

Fig. 21. Natural time course of frequency changes on the left side in 12 patients without surgery following SAH

SAH - NO ANEURYSM

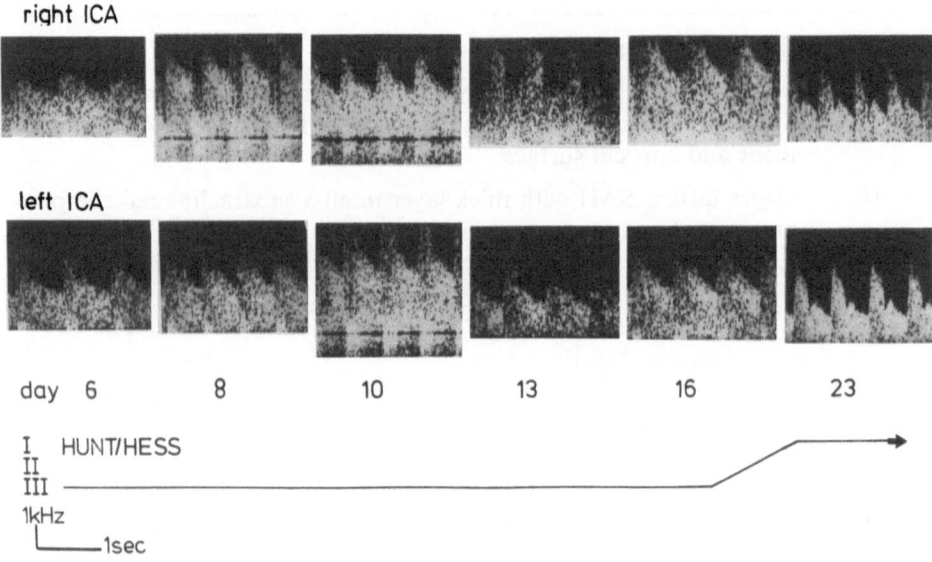

Fig. 22. Up to day 14 there is an increase in the flow velocities in the arteries, more in the right ICA than in the left, after which the frequency spectra slowly return to normal. On day 8 musical murmurs in the right ICA; on day 10 there is accumulation of low frequencies above and below the zero line as a sign of high velocities

In the patients in whom the Doppler frequencies increased to above 3 kHz, an aneurysm could be established as the cause of the subarachnoid hemorrhage in 5 cases (71%). Among the patients with frequencies of 3 kHz and less, an aneurysm could only be proved to be the cause of the SAH in one case (20%). The dependence of the increase in frequency on the severity of the SAH is illustrated in Figs. 23 a and b.

To what extent the natural course of the Doppler frequency after subarachnoid hemorrhage can be affected by early or delayed aneurysm surgery is discussed in the next chapters.

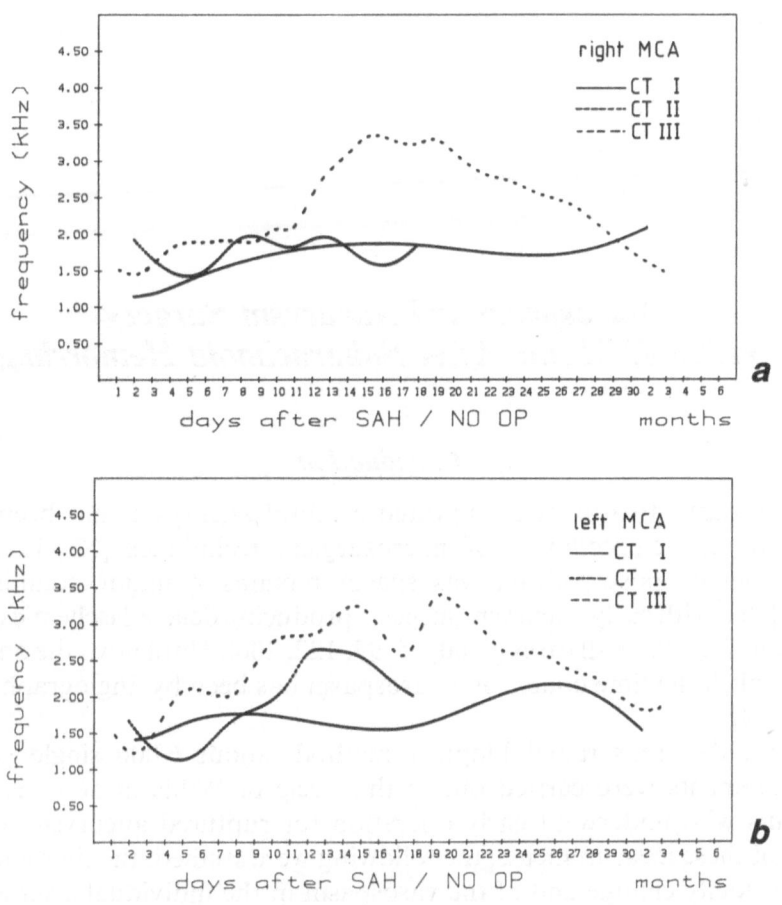

Figs. 23 a and b. Only patients with severe SAH (CT grade 3) show frequency increase due to vasospasm

Vasospasm and Aneurysm Surgery
Within 72 Hours After Subarachnoid Hemorrhage

Introduction

The operative treatment of ruptured cerebral aneurysms has been made safer by the employment of microsurgical techniques [12, 121, 212]. Nevertheless, postoperative vasospasm remains a major complication associated with early aneurysm surgery, producing delayed ischemic deficits in about 2–20% of all cases [4, 60, 75, 97, 122, 206]. Until now, the only way to establish the time course of a vasospasm has been by angiography [103, 173, 204].

With the transcranial Doppler method, about 6,000 single velocity measurements were carried out in the circle of Willis in 50 consecutive patients who underwent early operation for ruptured aneurysm. On the basis of these measurements, the following were studied: the time course of each velocity change and of the vasospasm in the individual arteries after SAH; the reaction to the origin of the hemorrhage; the frequency change on the side contralateral to the ruptured aneurysm; the effect of washing out clots from the subarachnoid space; the effect of preventive therapy with the calcium channel blocker, nimodipine; the use of transcranial Doppler sonography to improve postoperative therapy in order to minimize the incidence of delayed ischemic deficits (DIDs).

Patients

Fifty consecutive patients (27 women, 23 men) were operated on within 72 hours after a single SAH, which had been confirmed by lumbar puncture and computed tomography, or both. 68% were operated on within 24 hours, 24% between 25 and 48 hours, and 8% between 49 and 72 hours after the last SAH. The locations of the aneurysms are listed in Table 4; CT grading of the SAH, is presented in Table 5 and the relation of the preoperative clinical grading (Hunt and Hess) to the severity of the SAH is shown in Table 6.

Table 4. Location of the aneurysm in the 50 patients who underwent early aneurysm surgery

Aneurysm location	No. of patient	%
ACoA	23	46
ACoP	4	8
MCA	13	26
ACA (A 2)	2	4
AChorA	2	4
ICA Bif	3	6
Multiple	2	4
PICA	1	2

Table 5. Distribution of the different gradings in CT after SAH in the 50 patients

Grade		n	%
I	thin localized layer	2	4
II	thick layer in 2 of the 3 subarachnoidal compartments (basal cisterns, Sylvian fissures, interhemispheric space) or 1 subarachnoidal compartment and cortical surface	19	38
III	severe diffuse SAH with thick layers in all 3 subarachnoidal compartments or 2 and cortical surface	29	58
	Total	50	100

Table 6. With an increase in the severity of the SAH shown in CT, the clinical preoperative grade (Hunt and Hess) deteriorates

Hunt/Hess	Severity of SAH		
	I	II	III
I	1 (2)	2 (4)	0 (0)
II	1 (2)	10 (20)	4 (8)
III	0 (0)	6 (12)	15 (30)
IV	0 (0)	1 (2)	10 (20)

In all of the patients, nimodipine was intraoperatively applied to the exposed cerebral vessels to dilate the arterial vasospasm resulting from operative manipulations [13]. Nimodipine was then administered intravenously for 14 days (2 mg/h) and orally for another 6 days (4 × 60 mg) [4, 99, 122]. This schedule could be strictly adhered to in 33 patients, while in the others there was a difference of about 1 to 3 days. The balance of the circulating blood volume and red blood cell volume [97, 107, 161, 187] was carefully observed. Increased experience in assessing the transcranial Doppler findings aided in initiating prophylactic hypertension therapy for delayed ishemic deficits (DIDs) more effectively in order to obtain sufficient perfusion pressure for the brain.

Results

Vasospasm Within 72 Hours After the Last SAH

In 50 patients there were no angiographic signs of vasospasm during the first 72 hours after aneurysmal SAH. On the contrary, the vessels even appeared dilated (Figs. 24 and 25). The transcranial Doppler recordings showed no increased velocities that would correspond to vessel narrowing [62, 80].

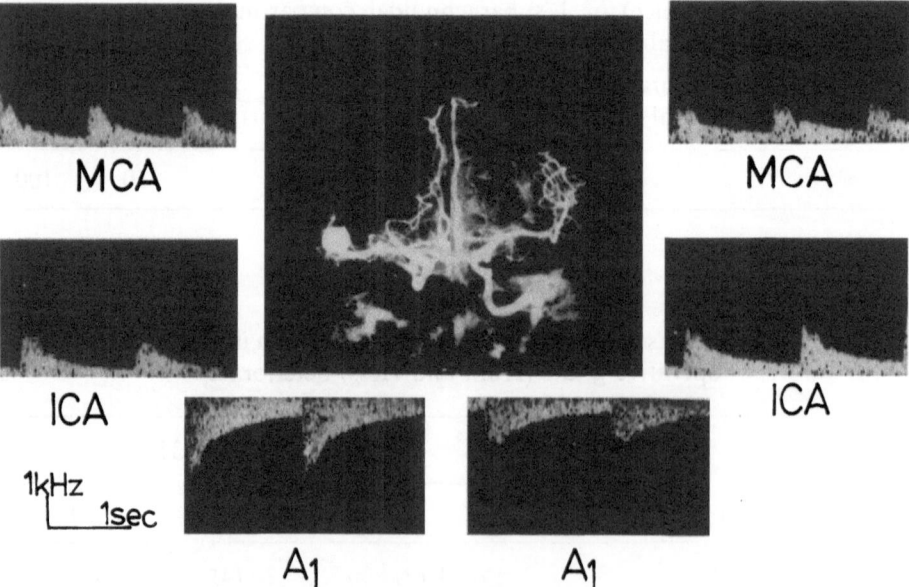

Fig. 24. Angiography and flow pattern in the different arteries 12 hours after SAH: angiographically no signs of vasospasm, the arteries even seem dilated. The Doppler frequencies are in the normal range

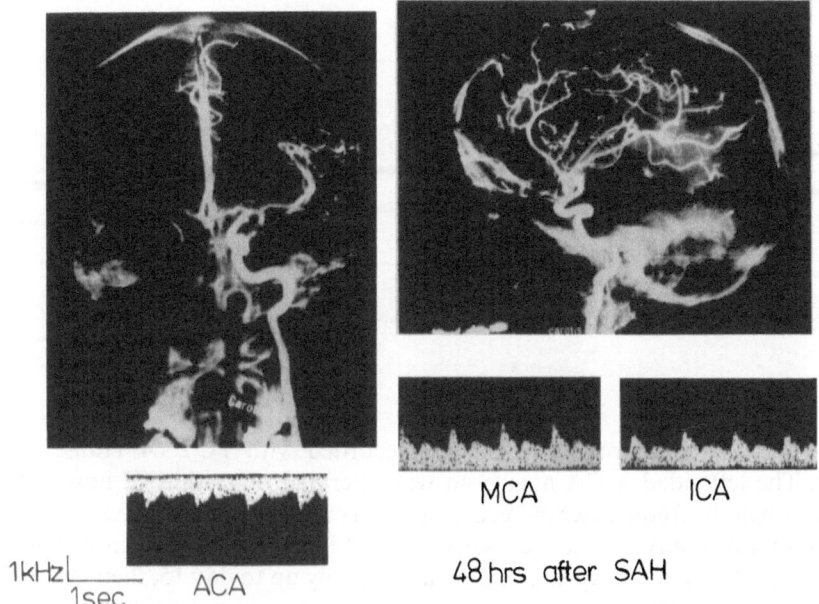

Fig. 25. 48 hours after SAH from ACoA aneurysm, angiography still shows no vasospasm, transcranial Doppler frequencies and flow patterns are normal

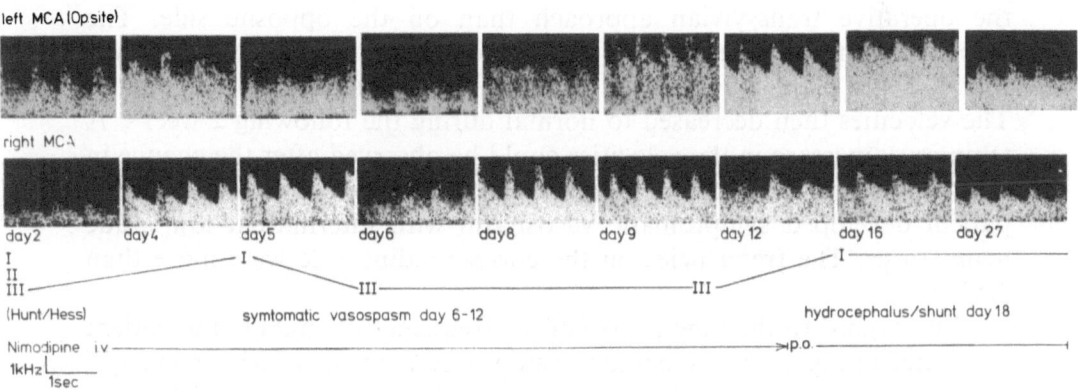

Fig. 26. Time course of frequency changes in both MCAs after early operation and nimodipine treatment. Severe frequency increase in the left MCA resulting from symptomatic vasospasm with delayed ischemic deficit from day 6 to day 1. Moderate (subcritical) vasospasm of the contralateral MCA. In both arteries there is frequency acceleration (day 16) after the change from intravenous to oral nimodipine administration

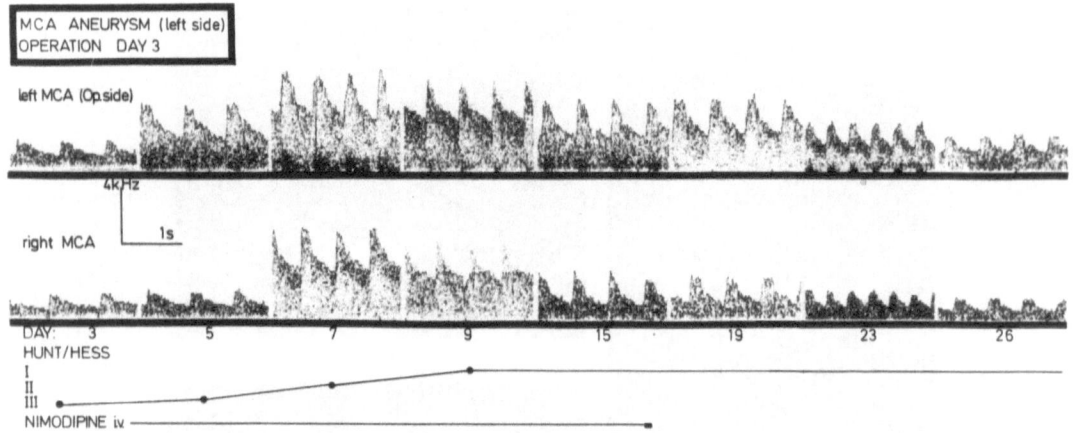

Fig. 27. Time course of frequency changes recorded with TC 2–64 Transcranial Doppler. The left-sided MCA aneurysm was operated on within 72 hours after SAH. Although the frequencies increased up to day 10, the clinical status improved continuously up to day 9. The frequencies were higher on the side on which the Sylvian fissure was split. Frequencies decreased slowly up to day 15, then increased from day 15 to day 19 after intravenous administration of nimodipine had been discontinued

Vasospasm Between Day 4 and Day 31 After SAH

Individual Cases

With regard to the time course of the frequency changes in the middle cerebral arteries, the typical velocity changes can be demonstrated by the following single example (Fig. 26): the velocities were higher on the side of the operative transsylvian approach than on the opposite side. The velocities increased during the period from day 4 to day 8, which was followed by a plateau phase with maximum velocities from day 9 to day 18. The velocities then decreased to normal during the following 2 weeks. A temporary increase in the velocities could be observed after the change in nimodipine application from intravenous to oral. Between day 6 and 12, the patient developed symptomatic vasospasm with intermittent low grade hemiparesis. The frequencies on the corresponding side were more than 3.5 kHz.

With regard to the time course of the frequency changes in the patient illustrated in Fig. 27, the maximum systolic frequency was 7.8 kHz on day 7 (3.2 times the normal), which corresponds to a velocity of 310 cm/sec (11.2 km/h). This patient, however, did not develop DIDs, and although the frequency increased as a result of vasospasm, the clinical condition improved from Hunt and Hess 3 to Hunt and Hess 1 by the 9th day after the SAH.

Further frequency courses are shown in Figs. 28 to 30.

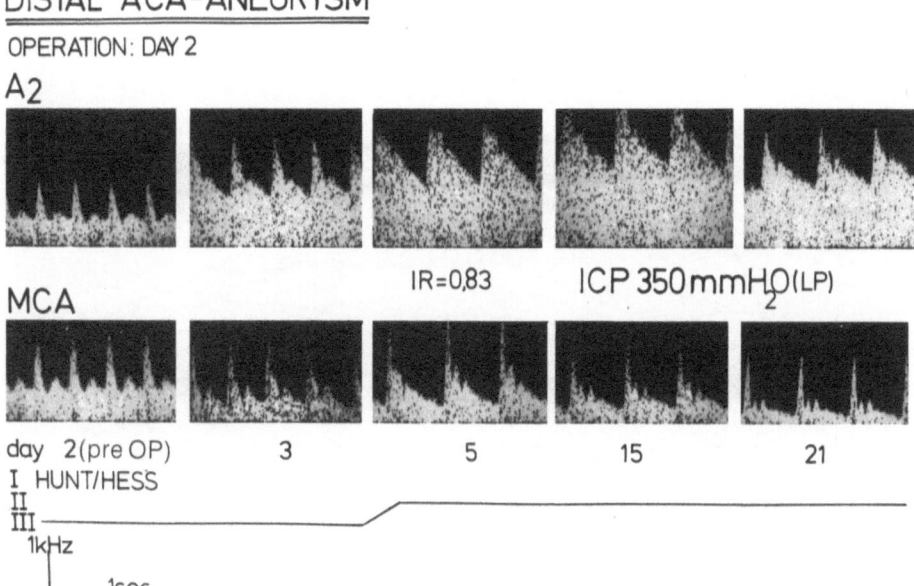

DISTAL ACA-ANEURYSM

OPERATION: DAY 2

A2

MCA

IR=0,83   ICP 350 mmH$_2$O(LP)

day   2(pre OP)   3   5   15   21
I HUNT/HESS
II
III
  1kHz
      1sec

Fig. 28. Subcritical vasospasm and moderate frequency increase up to day 15 in the pericallosal artery. The frequency spectrum of the MCA indicates increased peripheral vascular resistance due to hydrocephalus secondary to SAH. Improved clinical status up to day 5, even though frequency and index of resistance had increased

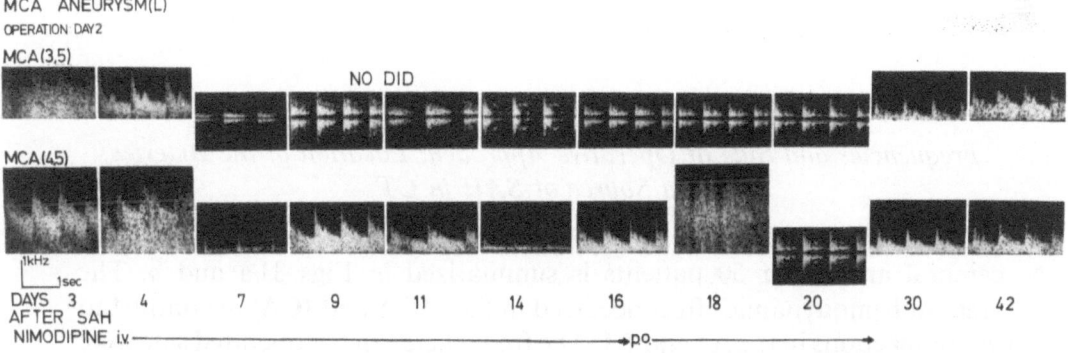

MCA ANEURYSM(L)

OPERATION DAY 2

MCA(3,5)   NO DID

MCA(4,5)

  1kHz
    1sec
DAYS 3   4   7   9   11   14   16   18   20   30   42
AFTER SAH
NIMODIPINE i.v.   p.o.

Fig. 29. Time course of frequency spectra in a 25-year-old man with subarachnoid hemorrhage and intracerebral temporal bleeding (preoperative status grade IV Hunt and Hess). In the distal part of the MCA (3.5) only such frequency phenomena as musical murmurs and bruits could be recorded, because the amount of erythrocytes in the presence of very high velocities is low and cannot be registered well with the Doppler instrument. Forty-two days after the SAH the Doppler frequencies were nearly normal. The patient developed no neurological symptoms

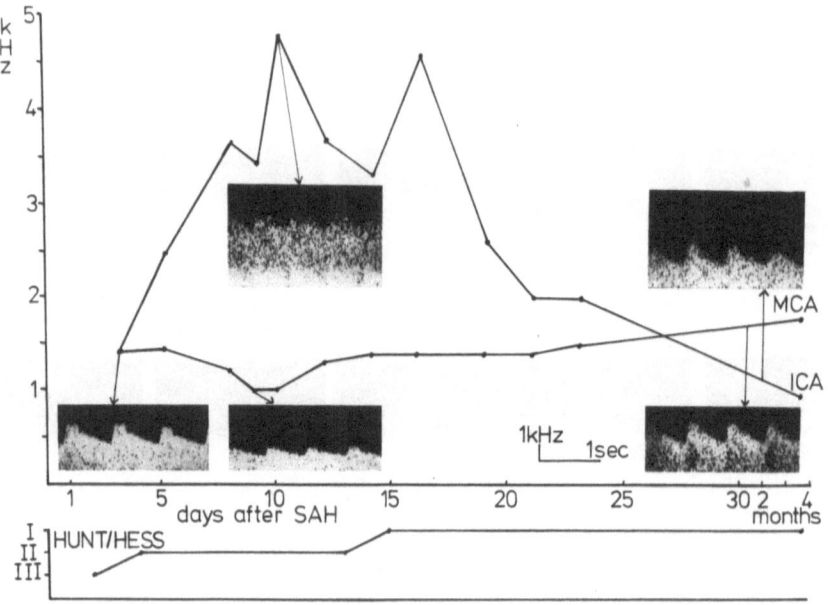

Fig. 30. This 34-year-old women suffered a subarachnoid hemorrhage and ACoA aneurysm. She had an older asymptomatic cervical occlusion of the internal carotid artery on the right side. When the vasospasm reached its maximum with increased velocities in the left ICA, the velocity in the contralateral MCA decreased. The vasospasm on the left side was critical because the collateral flow through the anterior communicating artery from the left to the right side had decreased. During treatment with hypertension there were no neurological deficits and the velocities in the MCA returned to normal very quickly

Frequencies and Side of Operative Approach, Location of the Arteries, and Source of SAH in CT

The time course of frequency changes due to vasospasm in the individual cerebral arteries of 50 patients is summarized in Figs. 31 a and b. The greatest hemodynamic effect occurred in the MCA and ICA, in contrast to minor reactions in the A1 and P1. The frequencies on the operated side were higher than on the contralateral side (Fig. 32). The extent of the post-operative increase in frequency has no direct relation to the pre-operative clinical condition of the patient (Fig. 33). Patients with severe hemorrhage and thick layers of blood in the subarachnoid space (CT III) developed more vasospasms than those with moderate or minor bleedings (CT II and I) (Figs. 34 a and b, 35 a–c, 36 a–c, 37 a and b).

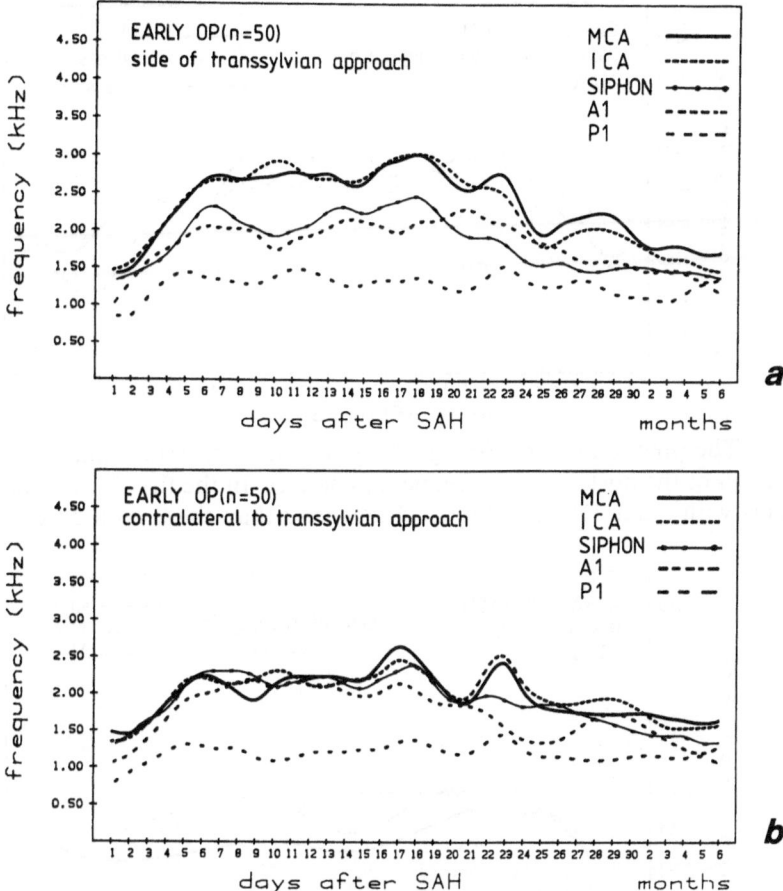

Figs. 31 a and b. Time course of frequency changes in the different arteries of the circle of Willis on the side of the operative approach (a) and the other side (b) in 50 patients. There is an increase in the first 10 days, then the maximum level is reached by days 18 and 19, after which there is a decrease

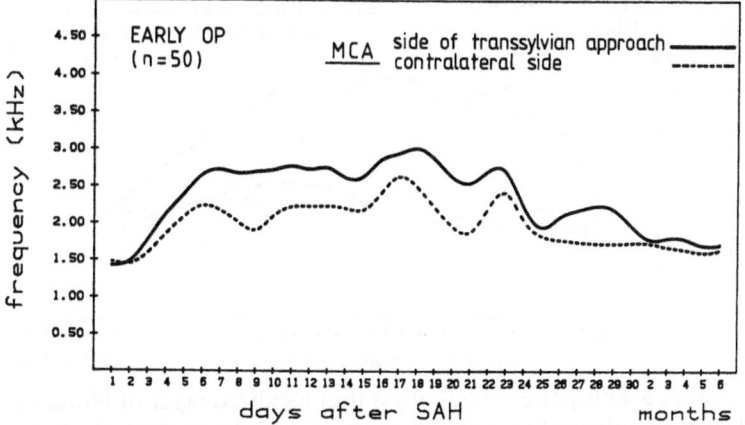

Fig. 32. The time course of frequency changes in the two MCAs after early aneurysm operation shows a higher velocity on the side of the operative approach. The difference is about 0.5 kHz (20 cm per second) between days 4 and 23

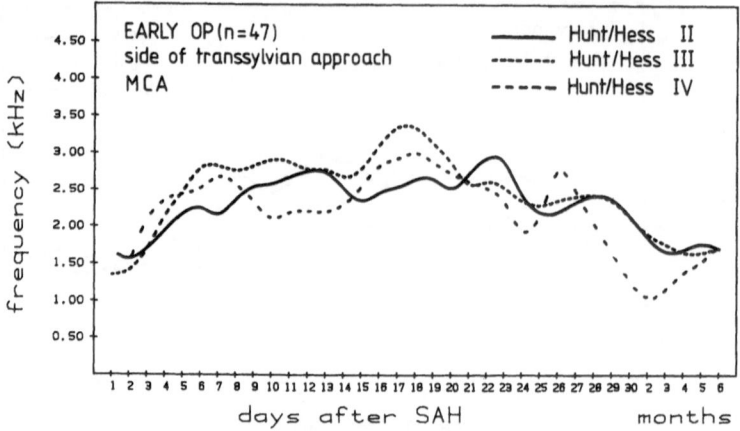

Fig. 33. The preoperative clinical grading according to Hunt and Hess gives no prediction of the postoperative frequency changes. In the first 20 days after SAH, patients with grade III show higher frequencies than those with grades II or IV

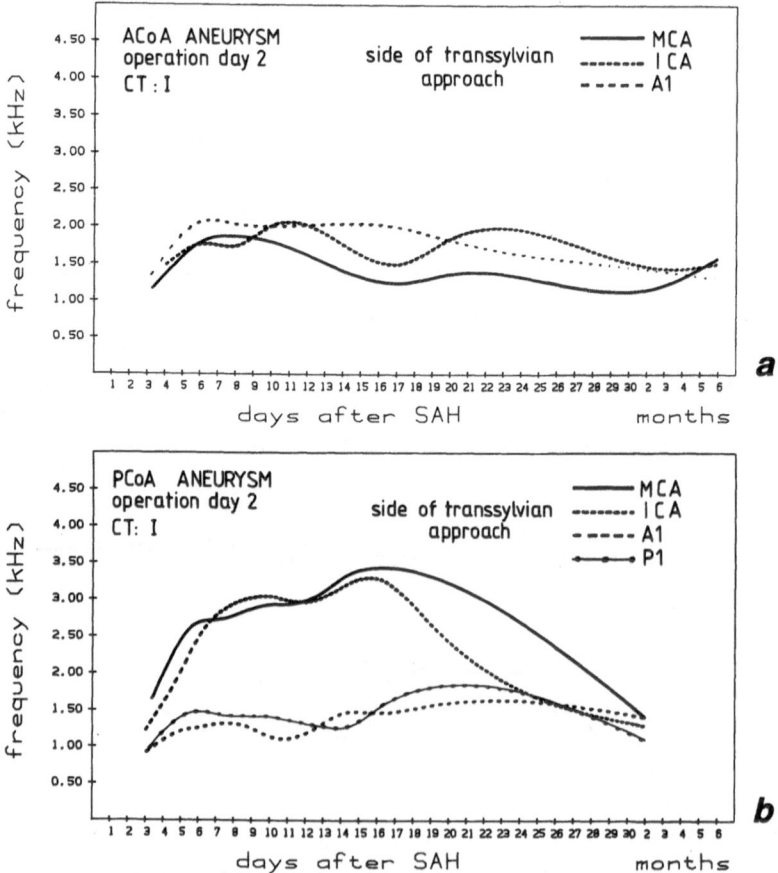

Figs. 34 a and b. *a* This patient had only a thin localized layer of blood in CT after SAH and showed only slight frequency changes. *b* In this patient, the frequencies in the MCA and ICA increased more than 3 kHz, even though he had only a thin localized layed of blood in CT

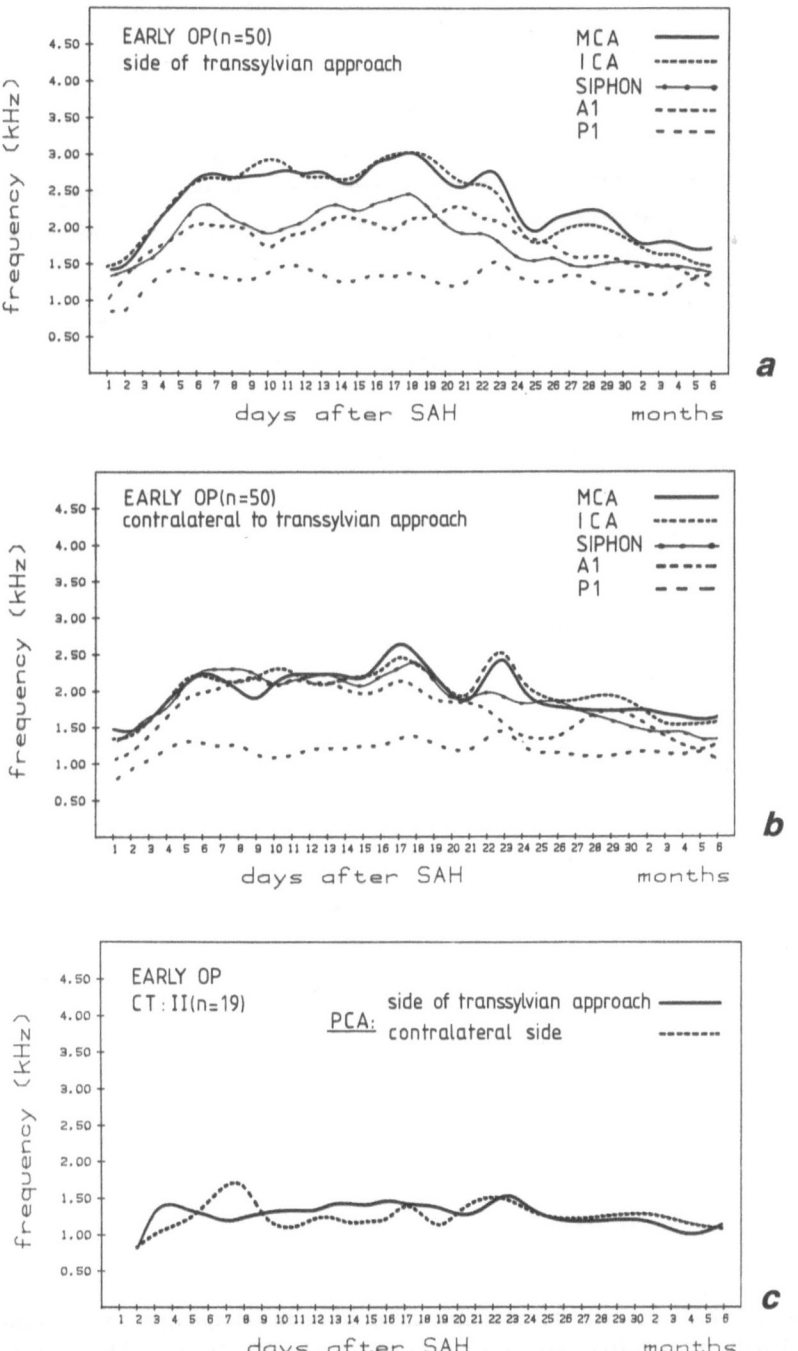

Figs. 35 a–c. When the source of the subarachnoid hemorrhage in CT was classified as grade 2, the frequency changes in the A1 (*b*) were less severe than in the MCA (*a*). In the posterior cerebral artery (*c*) there were hardly any significant frequency changes

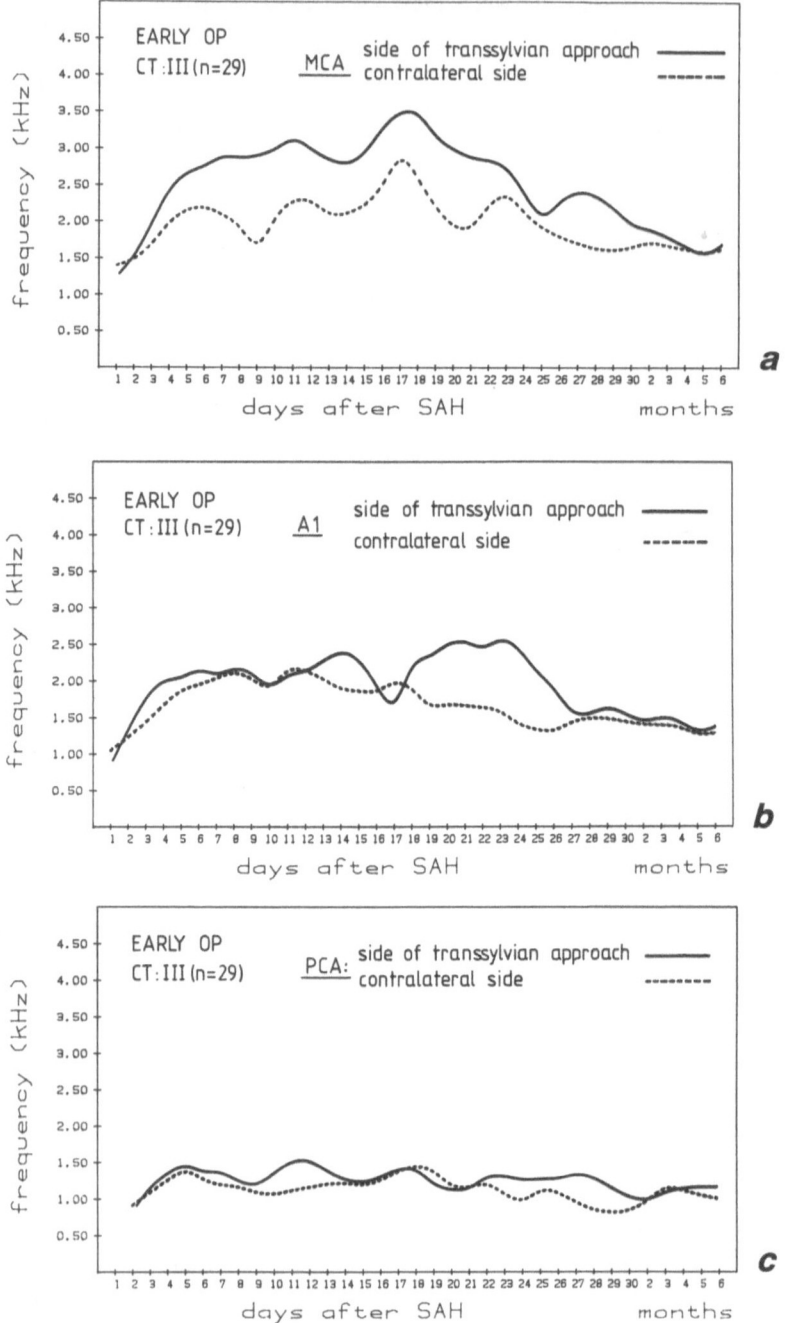

Figs. 36 a–c. Patients with severe subarachnoid hemorrhage in the CT classified as grade 3: *a* the highest frequency increase occurred in the MCA, and between the side of the operative approach and the contralateral side there was a difference of 1.2 kHz. *b* Increase and difference between sides was less in the A1 and *c* there was no statistically significant change in the posterior cerebral artery

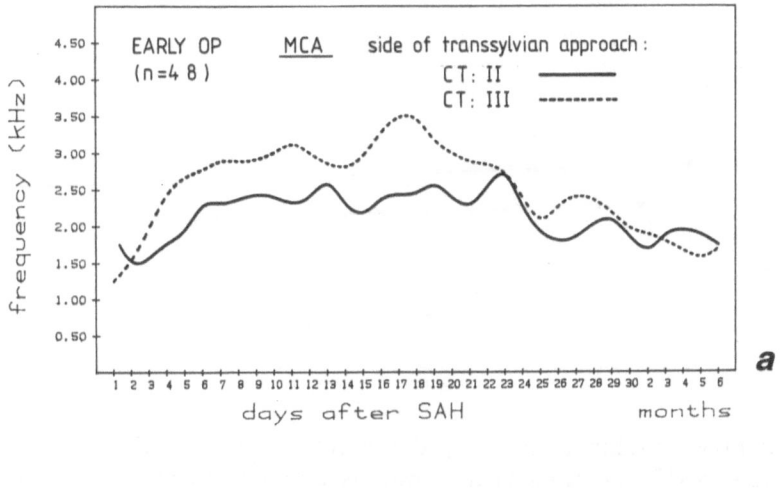

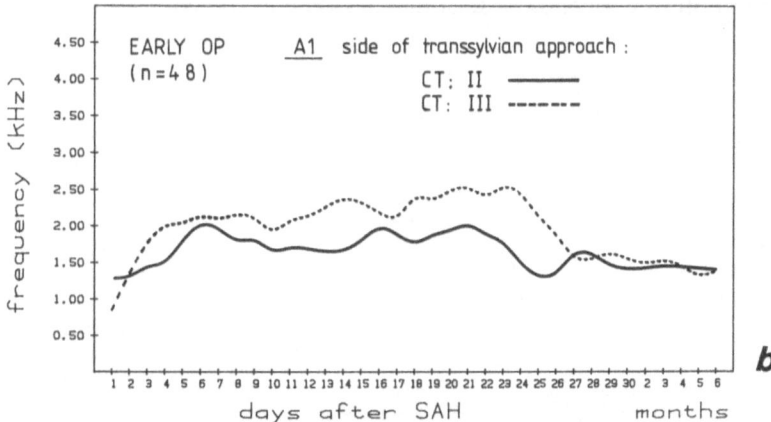

Figs. 37 a and b. The difference in frequency increase between the two sides depends on the maximum frequency reached after SAH. In the 48 patients the velocities were higher when CT showed severe subarachnoid hemorrhage (grade 3 as opposed to grade 2). In the MCA (*a*) this relationship was more pronounced than in the A1 (*b*)

Thirty three patients received nimodipine intravenously for exactly 14 days and orally for another 7 days. The mean and diastolic frequencies in the MCA (Fig. 38) on both the operated side and on the contralateral side

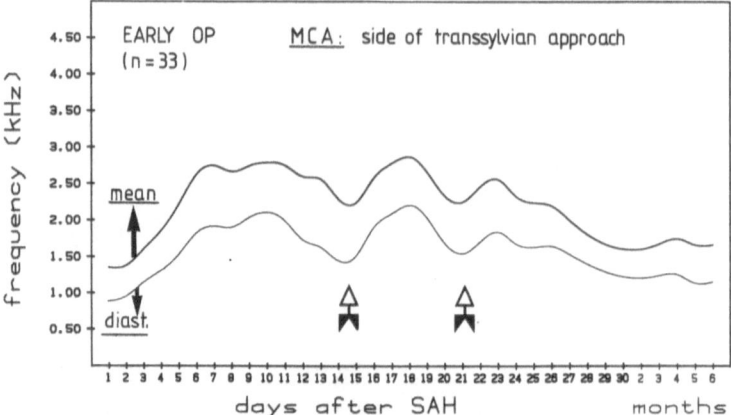

Fig. 38. After the nimodipine was changed from intravenous to oral administration on day 14 after SAH and the medication was discontinued on day 21, there was an increase in both the secondary diastolic and time averaged peak frequencies

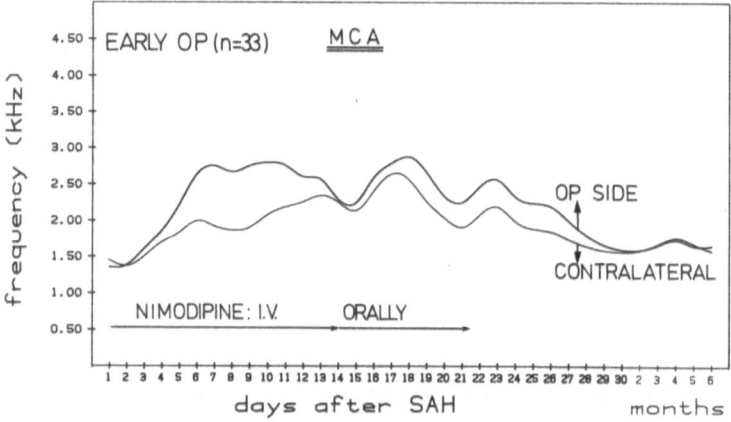

Fig. 39. In both MCAs the synchronous frequency changes demonstrate the nimodipine effect

(Fig. 39) increased temporarily after days 14 and 21. When nimodipine treatment was discontinued on the 16th day after SAH (Fig. 40), the frequencies increased again, whereas during preventive treatment with nimodipine there was a continuous drop of the frequencies. The changes in the frequency spectra induced by the application of nimodipine and by completion of the treatment are shown in Figs. 41 and 42).

Intracerebral Hemorrhage and Vasospasm

What is the effect of intracerebral hemorrhage following aneurysm rupture? A comparison of the frequency changes in the MCA on the operative side in

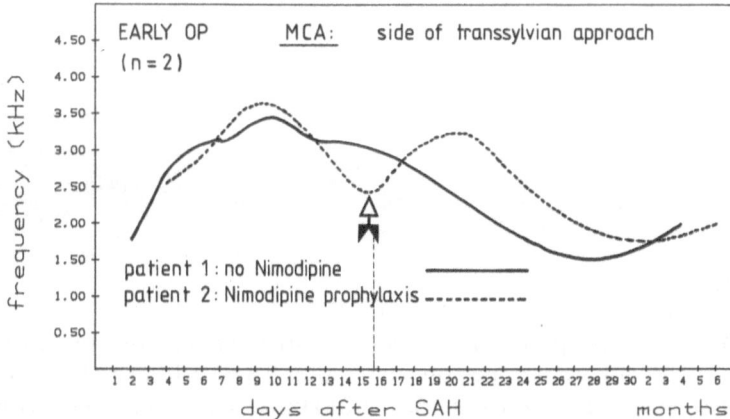

Fig. 40. Frequency changes in the MCA of 2 patients: patient 1 received no nimodipine prophylaxis. In the second patient the intravenous application was stopped on day 16 after SAH. Compared with the patients shown in Fig. 45, nimodipine was administered for 2 more days and the secondary increase in velocity occurred 2 days later

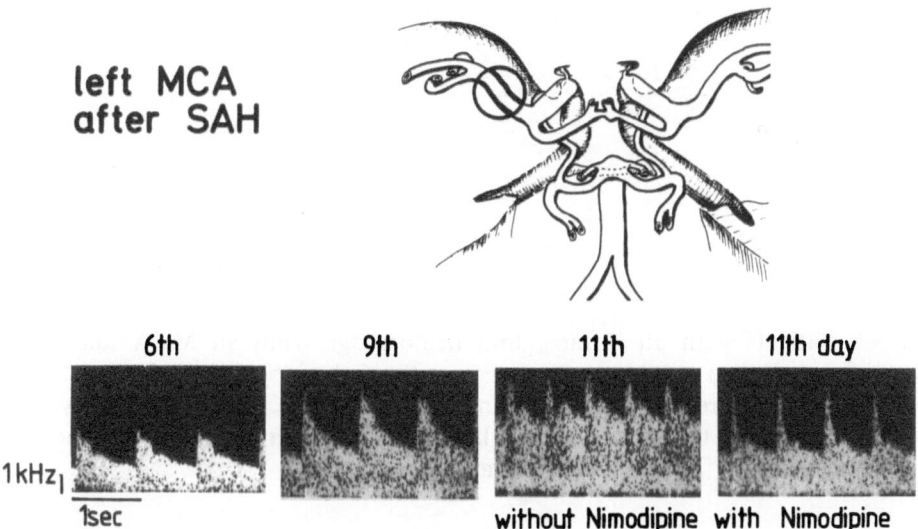

Fig. 41. Continuous velocity increase in the left MCA up to the 11th day after SAH without nimodipine prophylaxis. Six hours after intravenous application of nimodipine the velocity decreased considerably

eight patients operated on for aneurysm (Tab. 7) and intracerebral hematoma and those in 11 patients with severe SAH resulting from a midline aneurysm (ACoA) surprisingly showed that the time required for the maximum frequency to be reached differed by one week (Fig. 43).

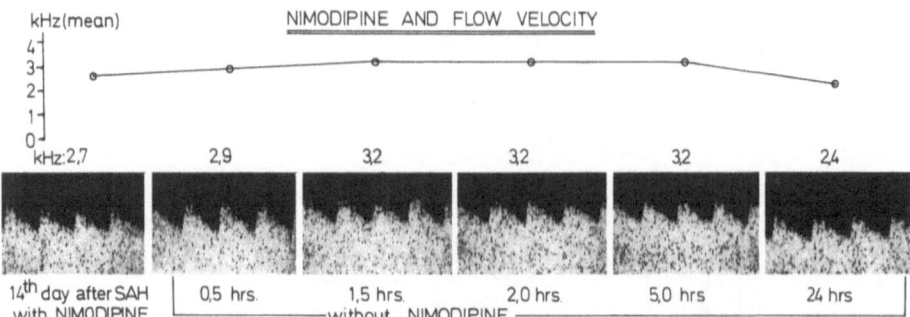

Fig. 42. The frequency spectra measured in short intervals after the intravenous nimodipine treatment was stopped on day 14 after SAH. Within an hour and a half the mean frequency increased from 2.7 to 3.2 kHz, which means a velocity increase of 20 cm per second

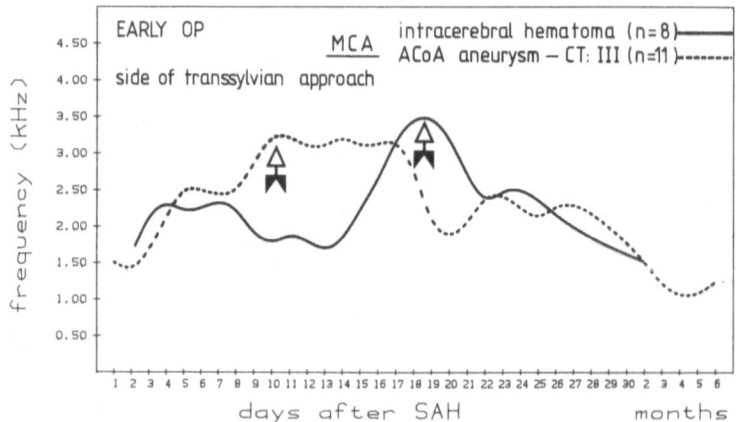

Fig. 43. Patients with an intracerebral hemorrhage from an MCA aneurysm surprisingly showed maximum frequency at the end of the 3rd week after SAH. Patients with severe SAH and midline aneurysms (*ACoA*) showed a typical constant increase in frequencies within the first 10 days with a maximum reached by day 17

Musical Murmurs in Transcranial Doppler Recordings

Musical murmurs as a sign of high blood velocity resulting in vessel wall vibration [3, 133, 191] could be recorded in 36% of the 50 patients (Table 8, Fig. 44). Such murmurs could be recorded more and more with increasing experience with the Doppler instrument. Fig. 45 shows this phenomenon not only in transcranial Doppler sonography, but also in intraoperative microvascular Doppler (20 MHz).

Table 7. Eight patients who suffered intracerebral and/or intraventricular hematoma due to aneurysm rupture

Patient	Aneurysm	CT	Hunt/Hess	Hematomas: cisternal and intracerebral	Intra-ventricular hematoma
m 25	MCA	II	IV	temporal	–
m 44	ACoA	III	III	frontal	+
m 39	ACA dist.	II	III	frontal	+
f 47	MCA	III	IV	temporal + Sylvian fissure	–
m 70	MCA	III	IV	temporal	–
f 59	MCA	III	IV	temporal	–
f 51	MCA	III	IV	temporal	+
m 66	ACoA	III	III	–	+

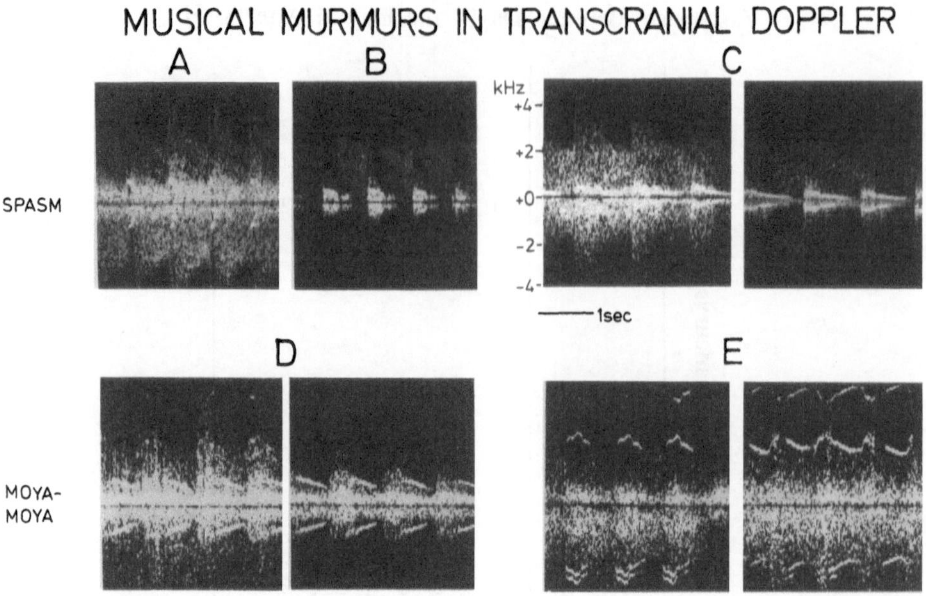

MUSICAL MURMURS IN TRANSCRANIAL DOPPLER

Fig. 44. Different types of musical murmurs and spasm and in high grade ICA stenosis. The higher the pure tones, the higher the blood flow velocities

Table 8. Onset and duration of musical murmurs and their location in 36% of the patients with SAH and early aneurysm surgery

Pat.	Aneurysm	Location of MM	Occurrence of MM (days after SAH)	Recording days
f 37	ICA (L)	MCA/ICA (L)	8	5
m 25	MCA (L)	MCA (L)	8	16
f 53	MCA (R)	MCA/ICA (R)	5	6
f 47	MCA (R)	MCA (R)	10	3
f 54	ACoA (r)	MCA/ICA (R)	12	1
m 34	ACoA (r)	MCA/ICA (R)	6	18
f 56	ACoA (r)	MCA (R)	~ 5 weeks	
		ACoA (A 1) (L)		
m 70	MCA (R)	MCA (R)	4	19
f 59	MCA (L)	MCA (L)	6	3
m 28	ACoA (1)	MCA/ICA (L)	6	4
m 45	PCoA (R)	MCA/ICA/A 1 (R)	7	2
f 65	PCoA (R)	MCA (R)	7	2
m 22	ICA (R)	MCA/ICA/A 1 (R)	8	12
f 38	PICA (L)	ICA (R)	11	2
m 51	MCA (R)	ICA (L)	6	1
f 39	ACoA (r)	ICA (R)	10	1
f 34	PCoA (L)	ICA/A 1 (L)	6	2
f 54	ICA (R)	ICA (L)	14	2

R/L = Location of aneurysm; r/l = Side of operative approach

MUSICAL MURMURS IN ICA
18th DAY AFTER SAH

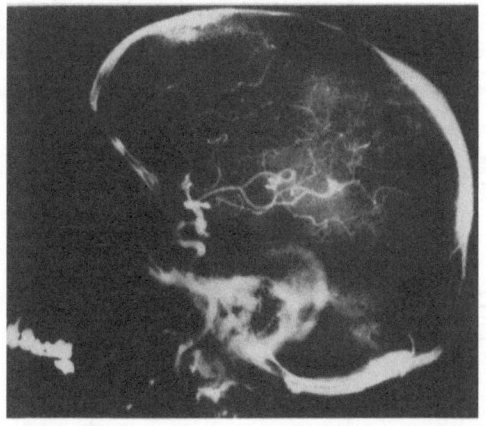

1kHz

1sec

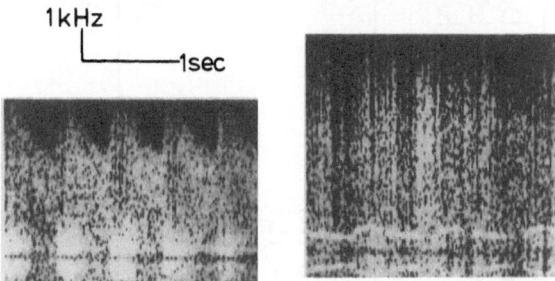

TRANSCRANIAL(2MHZ) – INTRAOPERATIVE(20MHZ)
DOPPLER

Fig. 45. 18 days after SAH from the posterior communicating artery aneurysm. There was a moderate stenosis of the proximal intracranial carotid artery. Intraoperative Doppler reveals moderate acceleration, but also musical murmurs as a sign of arterial wall vibrations. The transcranial Doppler findings of the same patient show local acceleration in the internal carotid artery and musical murmurs

Early Operation and DID

Among the first 16 patients in our series, seven developed delayed ischemic deficits, which improved without leaving permanent functional deficits (Table 9). All seven patients displayed a rapid increase in the velocities above 3 kHz between day 3 and day 4. DIDs occurred between day 6 and 12, while the Doppler frequencies in the MCA and the ICA were above 3.5 kHz (Fig. 46).

Based on the above results, we categorized the Doppler frequencies during vasospasm for clinical practice as follows (Table 10): a slight acceleration up to 2 kHz was in the normal range and was never observed in

Table 9. Data from the seven patients who suffered transient delayed ischemic deficits due to vasospasm. One patient died of cerebral infarction due to an unintentional decrease of perfusion pressure during vasospasm

Pat.	Aneurysm	Pre-op. CT	HUNT/ HESS	Symptomatic vessel	Days after SAH	DID days	MM days after SAH	Outcome
f 27	PCoA (R)	III	III	MCA (R)	9	3	0	good
f 63	ACoA (r)	III	III	MCA (R)	7	9	0	good
f 54	ACoA (l)	III	III	MCA (L)	12	2	12–13	good
f 52	PCoA (R)	II	II	MCA/ICA (R)	8	3	0	good
m 45	MCA (R)	II	III	MCA (R)	8	14	0	good
f 37	ICABif (L)	III	III	MCA/ICA (L)	7	2	8–13	good
f 43	MCA (L)	II	III	MCA (L)	13	3	0	good
f 45	ACoA (r)	III	II	MCA/ICA (r)	12	1		dead (RR-management)

R/L = location of aneurysm; r/l = operative approach; mortality 2%; transient DID 14%.

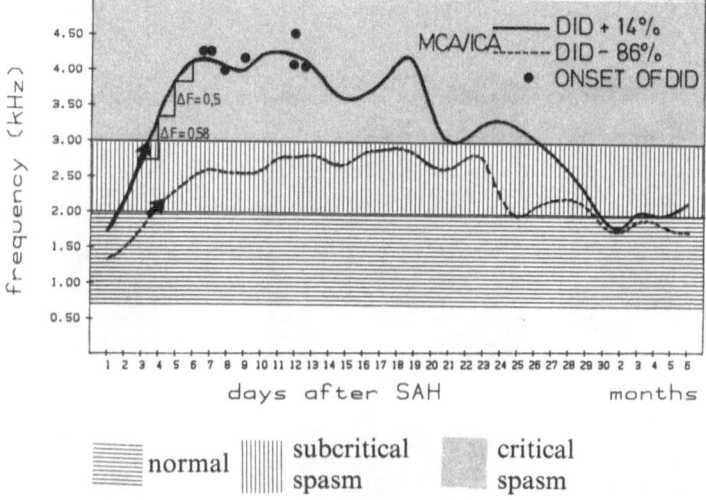

Fig. 46. A rapid frequency increase in the first 6 days to more than 3.5 kHz indicates an extreme risk for the patient. The points represent the onset of DID in the 7 patients. The time averaged peak frequencies of the other patients never exceeded 3.0 kHz and showed a slow increase in the first 6 days. Frequency ranges are therefore categorized as follows: up to 2 kHz is considered normal, frequencies between 2 and 3 kHz represent subcritical spasm, and above 3 kHz denote critical spasm

Table 10. Flow pattern, blood flow velocity, and their clinical significance in patients suffering SAH

Range of velocities	Doppler frequency* (kHz)	Flow pattern	Clinical importance
Normal	≤ 2	normal laminar	
Unspecific acceleration	~ 2	normal laminar	must be controlled
Subcritical spasm	2–3	normal laminar perhaps turbulent and bruits	preventive therapy
Critical spasm	≥ 3	irregularities, wall artefacts, bruits, musical murmurs	symptomatic therapy

* Time averaged peak frequency.

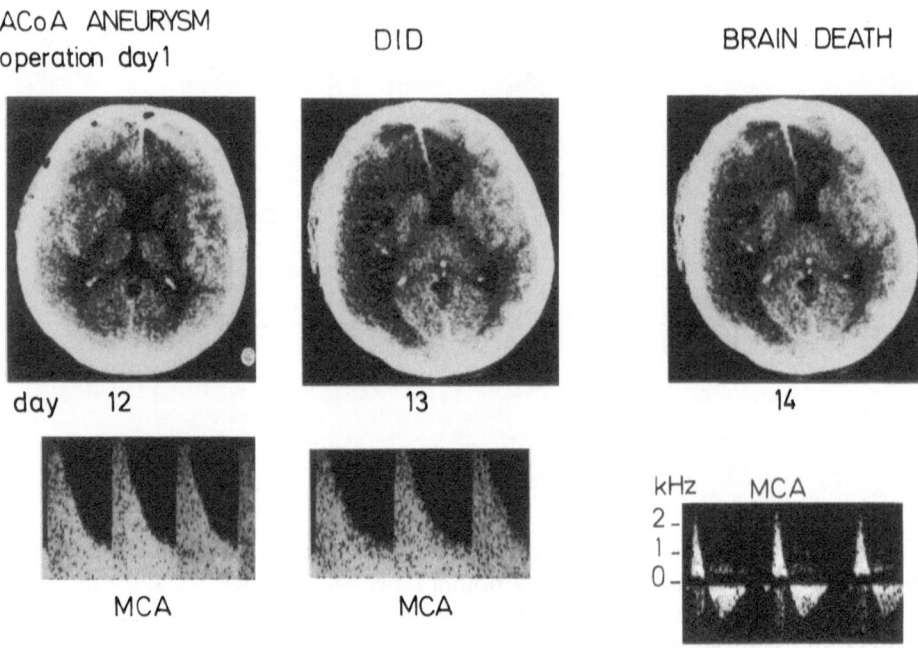

Fig. 47. This patient recovered well up to day 12 after the acute aneurysm operation. Then on day 13 she developed a delayed epidural hematoma, which was treated surgically. Following the operation she suffered unintentional hypertension for 2 hours. On the next day she was comatose, showed brain infarction in the CT, and the flow pattern in the MCA was reverberating, indicating zero net flow

angiographically confirmed vasospasm. Frequencies between 2 and 3 kHz were termed "subcritical". These velocities were registered in those patients who did not develop ischemic deficits. Frequencies higher than 3 kHz denote critical vasospasm, since all of the patients who developed symptoms were in this group.

Clincal Outcome

The Degree of Disability According to the Glasgow Outcome Scale

One patient (2%) died as a result of unintentionally lowered blood pressure during severe vasospasm (Fig. 47). Two patients (4%) were severely disabled, six patients (12%) were moderately disabled, and 41 patients (82%) were able to lead a full and self-sufficient life.

Discussion

For the investigation of the time course of the blood flow velocities, the different arteries have to be recorded at the same depth and with the same angle between the ultrasonic beam and the artery. The latter can be achieved by adjusting the insonation angle to show the highest Doppler shift.

When the arteries are narrowed, the blood flow velocity increases. The compensatory frequency acceleration can be measured by TCD, which shows vessel narrowing earlier than angiography, since the velocity increase is proportional to the second power of the diameter reduction.

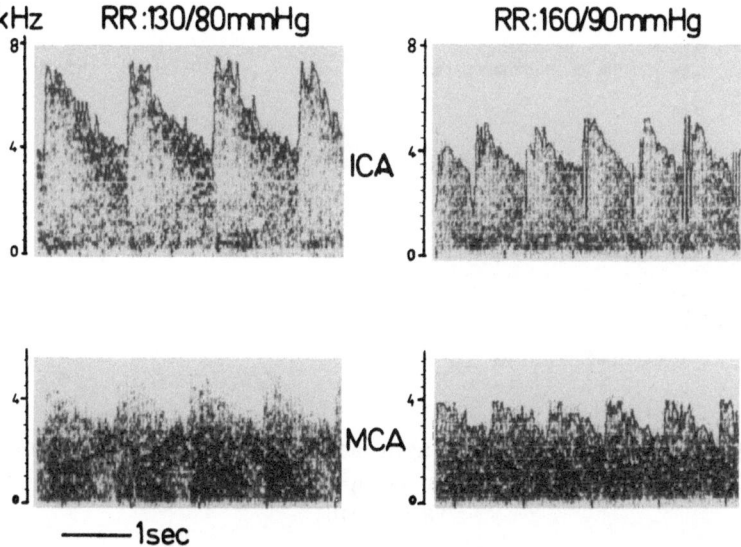

Fig. 48. Frequency spectra before and after the blood pressure was increased. There is a reduction of the frequencies in the ICA after induced hypertension

In the first 72 hours after SAH, we did not observe accelerations as a sign of vasospasm. After 72 hours, a more or less rapid velocity increase begins and continues from day 4 to 10. The maximum is reached between day 10 and 20, after which the velocities decrease. These findings correlate with the CBF measurements [136], which indicate a decrease in the cerebral blood flow in the first 14 days after SAH. The patients with a rapid increase in the velocities in the first 6 days to more than 3.5 kHz may develope DIDs. When there is a daily frequency increase from day 3–7 after SAH of about 0.5 kHz, we term this the Doppler index of delayed ischemic deficits (DIDID) (Fig. 46). In such cases, we prefer preventive hypertension therapy, keeping systolic blood pressure between 130 and 150 mm Hg in normotensive patients and between 140 and 170 mm Hg in hypertensive patients. Increasing perfusion pressure by induced hypertension resulted in a reduction of the Doppler shift in the case shown in Fig. 48 [8].

The importance of the blood pressure for the cerebral perfusion pressure in vasospasm is illustrated by the history of one patient (Fig. 47): a 54 year old woman with an aneurysm in the anterior communicating artery was pre-operatively classified as grade 2 (Hunt and Hess), and CT showed a severe subarachnoid hemorrhage. The uneventful operation was performed within 24 hours after the bleeding. Between day 8 and 12 we treated the patient with induced hypertension because of vasospasm detected by Doppler so-

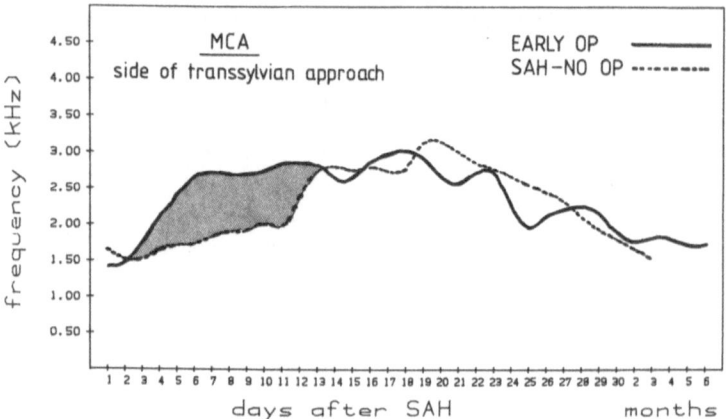

Fig. 49. On the side of the operative approach the time it takes for the maximum velocity to be reached is shorter in comparison with natural time course of vasospasm

nography (4 kHz in the MCA) and a slight hemiparesis on the left side. After a delayed epidural hematoma had been evacuated, a noninduced drop of the systolic blood pressure to 60 mm Hg occurred, which lasted two hours. After this, the patient became comatose and CT revealed an infarction of the right cerebral hemisphere. Transcranial Doppler showed a reverberat-ing flow pattern with a net zero flow as a typical sign of brain death.

The theory that washing out clots from the subarachnoid space diminishes the severity of the vasospasm could not be confirmed. In the region where the clots were removed, namely, on the side of the operative approach, the frequencies were always higher than on the opposite side. On day 11 or 12, the highest velocities were reached in both hemispheres, which may be due to the fact that the vasoconstrictive substances may have a faster and better effect on the cleaned vessels than on vessels with intact arachnoid sheets (Fig. 49). Knowing this we remove only as much subarachnoid blood as necessary for an adequate operative view.

The relationship between the severity of SAH and vasospasm, *i.e.,* the more blood, the more spasm, is clearly illustrated in Fig. 37 a. For the

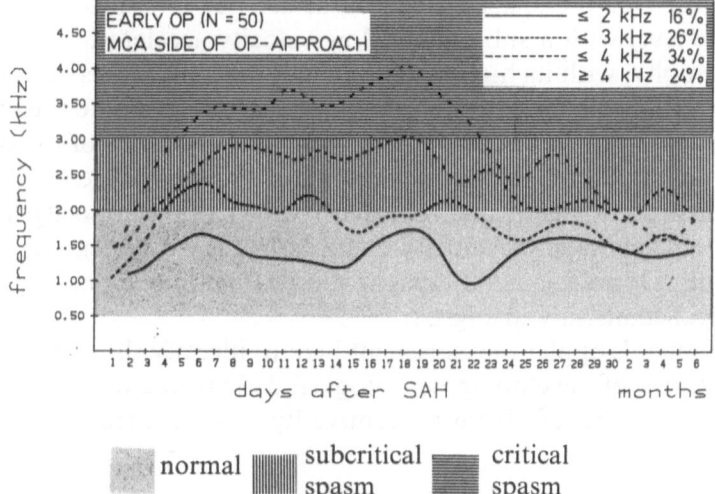

Fig. 50. Frequency range in 50 patients following acute aneurysm operation. Only 16 percent is in the normal range, while the other 84 percent shows moderate or severe frequency increase in the MCA on the side of the operative approach

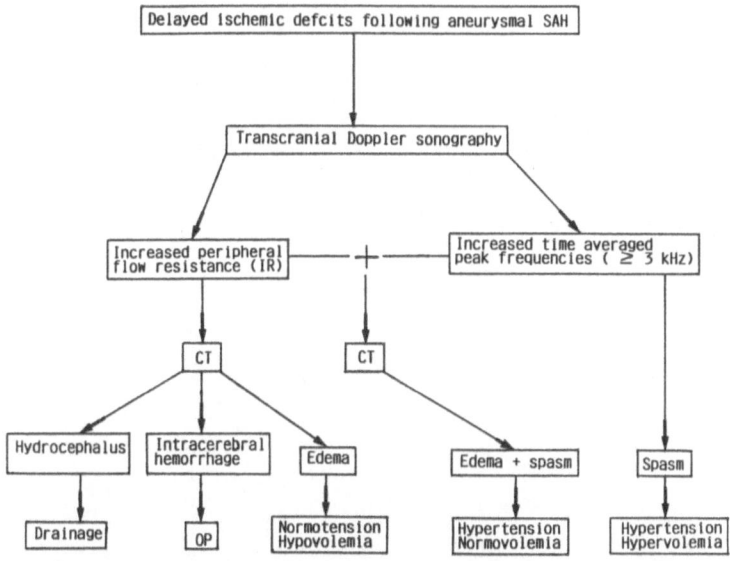

Fig. 51. The value of transcranial Doppler in the differential diagnosis of delayed ischemic deficits following aneurysmal SAH. Angiography is no longer necessary

second acceleration that results from changing the form of nimodipine administration, there are two possible explanations:

1. a lowered nimodipine level reduces the dilatation of the small resistance vessels, decreases the collateral flow, and induces higher flow velocities through the spastic arteries,

2. dilatation of the spastic large basal arteries is reduced by a lower nimodipine level with a subsequent flow velocity acceleration.

Angiography, with its high morbidity and mortality rates in the case of vasospasm [128, 129, 158], is no longer necessary to evaluate the existence and severity of this phenomenon. The individual reactions of the different arteries of the circle of Willis as a result of the subarachnoid hemorrhage can be followed atraumatically and repeatedly with Doppler velocity measurements. The percentage of velocity changes in the 50 patients is given in Fig. 50. The "Doppler-guided" diagnostic and therapeutic management is presented schematically in Fig. 51.

Transcranial Doppler measurement help to identify those patients who have a high risk of developing neurological deficits due to vasospasm and those who would benefit from preventive hypertensive treatment.

Correlation of Angiographically Confirmed Vasospasm and Stenosis with Transcranial Doppler

After the Doppler measurements had indicated the possible existence of vasospasm, angiography was performed only in a few cases, at which time high Doppler shifts were measured. The diameter of the cerebral arteries was measured by the split image focussing technique according to Huber and Handa [85] from the angiograms in eight patients with vasospasm who had undergone delayed aneurysm surgery. When the frequencies were plotted against the corresponding vessel diameters, an inverse correlation of frequency and diameter could be established for the MCA and ICA (Fig. 52). No clear correlation could be found in the A1. All of the eight patients with angiographically confirmed vasospasm had frequencies above 3 kHz.

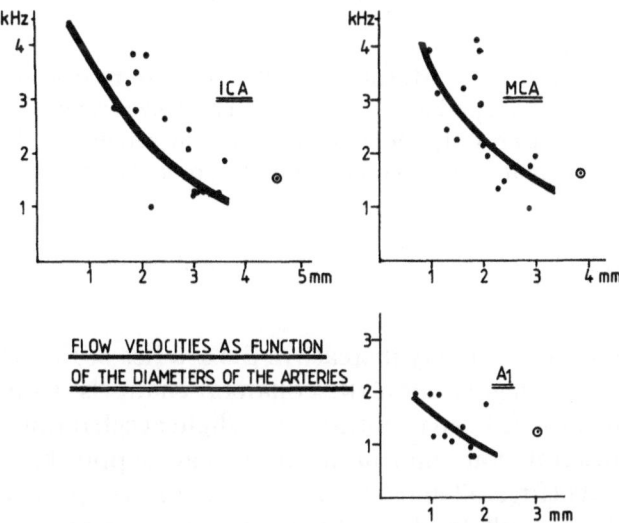

Fig. 52. Inverse relationship of vessel diameter and frequency in 8 patients with angiographically confirmed spasm. While this relationship is clearly shown in ICA and MCA, the frequency increase is much less in the A1 where there are many collaterals

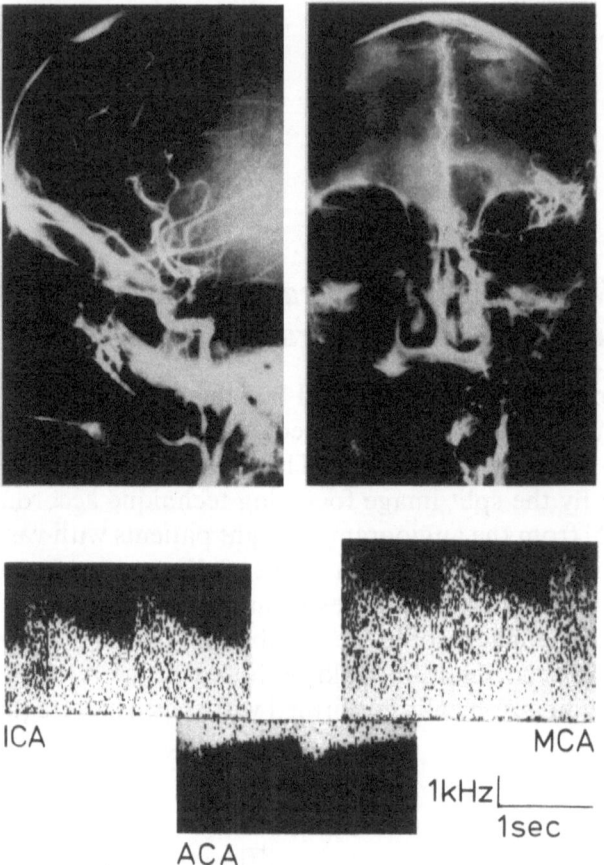

Fig. 53. 9th day after SAH. Morphologically, there is nearly identical lumen narrowing in the ICA, A1, and MCA. The velocity increase is highest in the MCA, however, because there are only few collaterals. In contrast, in the A1 the velocity is normal due to the large number of collaterals

The compensatory velocity increase in the arteries of the circle of Willis depends to a large degree upon the collateral channels. Consequently, a marked spasm of the A 1 can produce only a slight acceleration, since a well-functioning anterior communicating artery can supply blood from the contralateral side (Figs. 53 and 54). In contrast, severe spasm of the MCA, which has only few collaterals, will produce a pronounced acceleration.

Differentiation between vasospasm and clip-induced arterial stenosis or progressive localized arterial stenosis can be made atraumatically by using the transcranial Doppler method (Figs. 55–57).

SPASM 11th DAY AFTER SAH

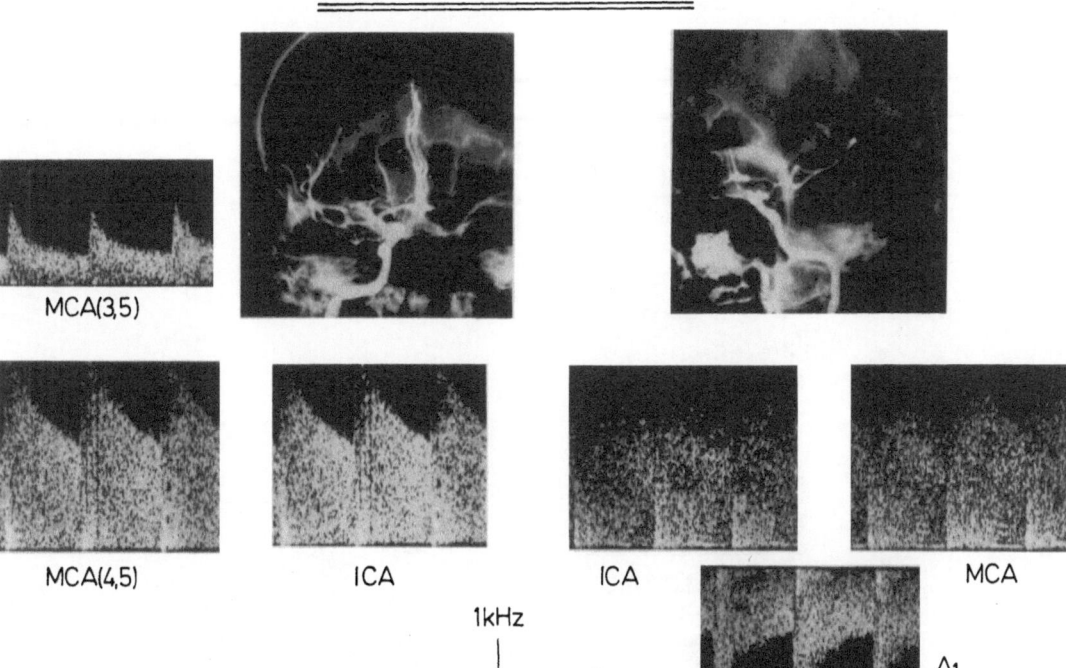

Fig. 54. 11th day after SAH. Angiographically, the spasm of the arteries on the right side is less severe than on the left. Transcranial Doppler shows the corresponding frequency spectra of these arteries

The relationship between the diameter of the vessel and the compensatory blood flow velocity was also established by Aaslid [2]. The time averaged peak frequencies in the ICA and MCA of 3–4 kHz, correspond to a vessel lumen of 1–2 mm. The frequency range of 2–3 kHz, which is categorized as "subcritical", corresponds to a vessel diameter of more than 2 mm. Doppler frequencies of 2 kHz correspond to a vessel diameter of approximately 3 mm.

The severity of vasospasm should not be clinically assessed by the absolute frequency increase alone. The high Doppler frequencies measured in all of the sections of the circle of Willis signify a higher risk of the patient developing ischemic deficits than localized high velocities.

On the basis of transcranial Doppler sonographic measurements, the timing of angiography and delayed aneurysm surgery (72 hours after SAH) can be selected so as to rule out the risk of performing angiography or surgery during a severe spasm.

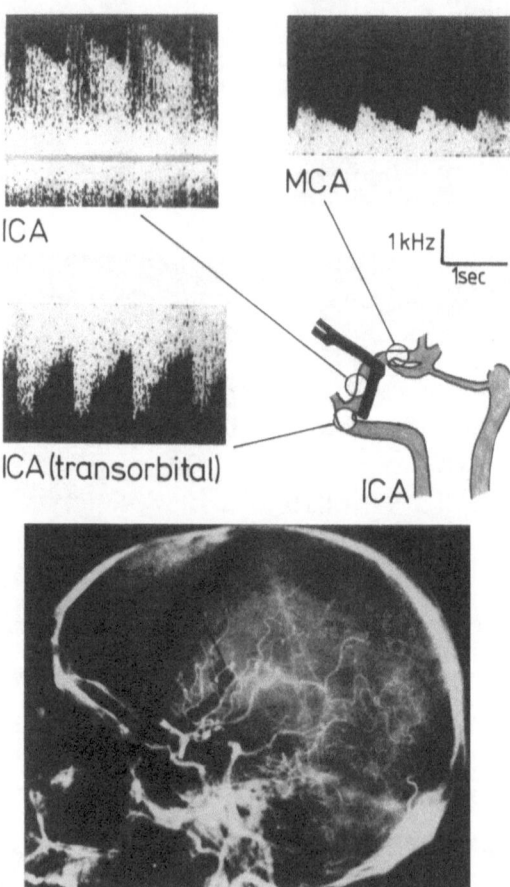

Fig. 55. Carotid ophthalmic aneurysm. Moderate reduction of the vessel caliber due to tight clip. Transcranial Doppler shows a corresponding localized acceleration of the internal carotid artery

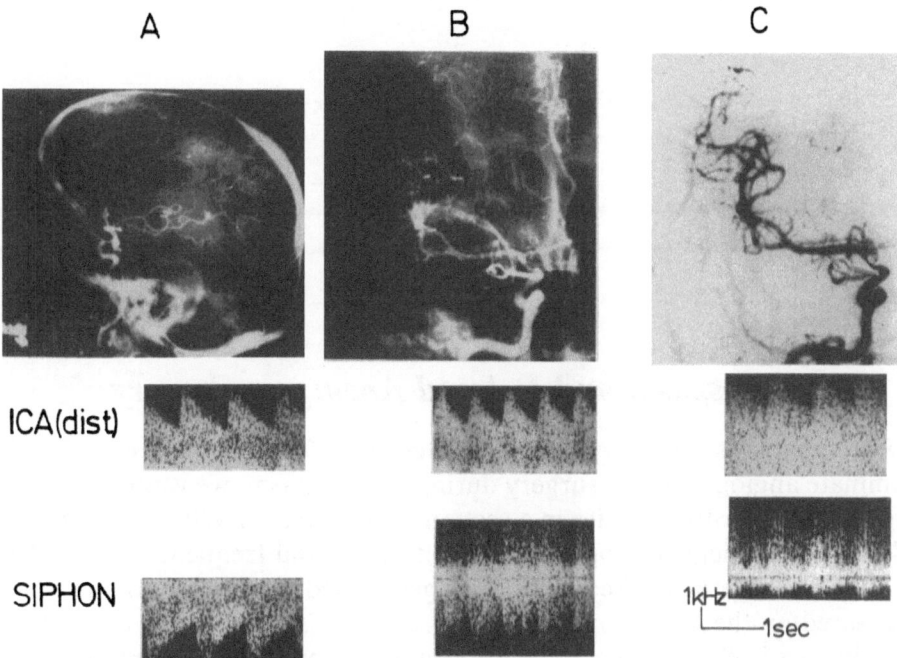

Fig. 56. Progressive stenosis of the supraclinoid portion of the internal carotid artery after clipping of a posterior communicating artery aneurysm on day 18 after SAH. *A* Increase in flow velocity according to the progression of the stenosis, *B* 6 weeks after the 1st angiography and, *C* 7 weeks later

MCA STENOSIS AND TRANSCRANIAL DOPPLER

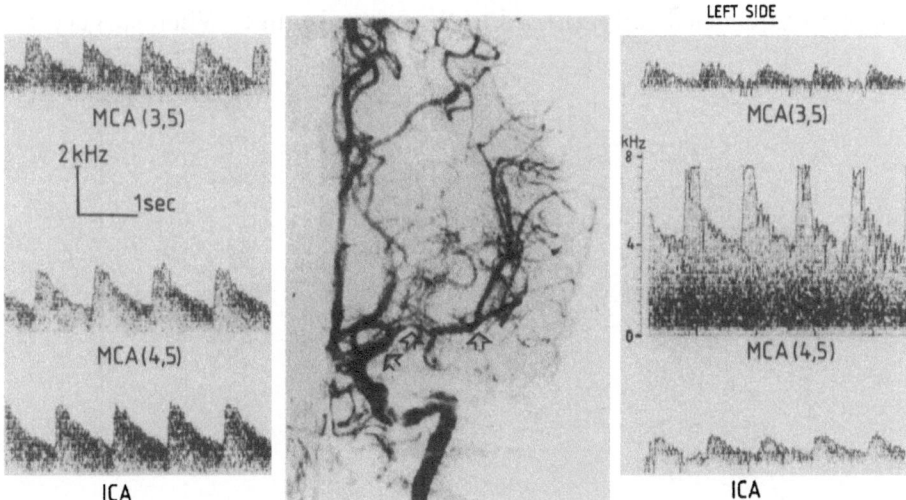

Fig. 57. In angiography there is a stenosis of the trunk of the MCA. Transcranial Doppler shows an increase in the velocity measured at a depth of 4.5 cm. Distally, the frequency spectrum shows reduced velocities and damped waveforms in comparison with the opposite side. Transcranial Doppler investigation is sufficient to follow up disease. Angiography is no longer necessary

Vasospasm and Delayed Aneurysm Surgery

Twenty patients were operated on later than 72 hours after SAH. To eliminate angiography or surgery during severe spasm, we waited until the highest Doppler frequencies in a section of the circle of Willis were around 3 kHz. One patient was operated on with an initial frequency of 3.4 kHz.

The postoperative frequency changes varied according to the value measured on the day of operation (Fig. 58). Fig. 59 shows one example of the changes in the frequency spectra resulting from delayed surgery on the 19th day after SAH.

The patients undergoing delayed aneurysm surgery also showed frequency changes, particularly on the side of the operative approach in the MCA and the ICA. Depending on the time of the SAH or of the operation, or both, the Doppler frequencies increased at different speeds and then slowly returned to normal. As a result of the operation, a further increase in frequency occurred within the first four weeks after the SAH, even when the Doppler frequencies had returned to the normal range. When surgery was

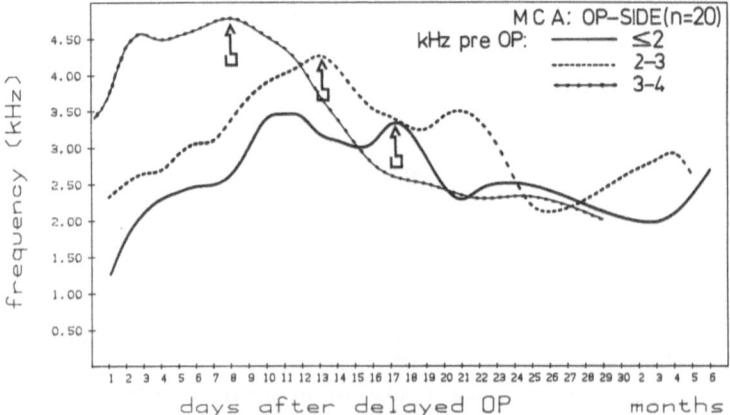

Fig. 58. Time course of frequency changes in 20 patients with delayed aneurysm surgery. The higher the initial frequencies, the earlier the decrease of the frequency begins, in accordance with the natural time course of vasospasm

performed while the Doppler frequencies were still high, *e.g.,* in the third week after the bleeding, the maximum frequency was reached more quickly and it returned to normal sooner than after early surgery.

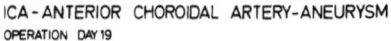

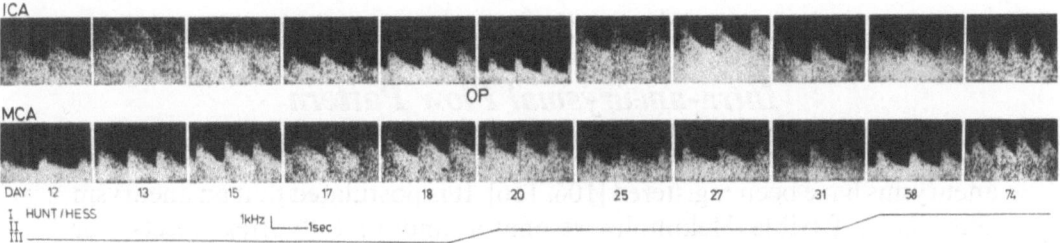

Fig. 59. Frequency changes before and after delayed aneurysm surgery in ICA and MCA. Near the aneurysm (*ICA*), velocities increased again after the operation. Even after 74 days following SAH, the velocities are twice the norm in ICA and MCA (vessel-wall?—hyperemia?)

It can thus be assumed that the natural time course of vasospasm is affected only temporarily and to various degrees by the operation. In 25% of the patients referred to our department three days after the SAH, surgery was delayed until the Doppler findings indicated the appropriate time for the operation. The following criteria were used to indicate surgery: when the maximum frequency had been exceeded; when a marked reduction of the spasm had been determined; and when the frequencies were below 3 kHz.

Intra-aneurysmal Flow Pattern

Using an electronic stethoscope, specific frequency patterns caused by aneurysms have been registered [106, 156]. It is postulated that an aneurysm acts like a flexible Helmholtz resonator and that "vortex sheets" or turbulence therefore occur.

In his intraoperative Doppler sonographic examinations on aneurysms, Nornes [151] found a clearly slower velocity than in the feeding arteries. The fact that whirlpool-like movements of the blood can be seen intraoperatively through thin walls does not necessarily mean that there is turbulent flow in the aneurysm.

Using a computer model, Austin [15] describes pressure and velocity changes in the aneurysm and in the feeding arteries. When the blood pressure is increased, the intra-aneurysmal pressure rises. The perfusion, however, does not. Raising the pulse frequency also raises the intra-aneurysmal pressure and diminishes the circulation in the aneurysm. When there is vasospasm distal from the aneurysm, the pressure in the aneurysm increases. Only 5% of the blood volume measured in the feeding arteries flows through the aneurysm. Pressure alterations are primarily responsible for the rupture of an aneurysm and not turbulent flow. In 1984 Hashimoto [81] detected turbulent flow mainly in broad-based aneurysms with little volume. Using a glass and silastic model, he found low velocities in the dome of the aneurysm in the Doppler sonographic recording.

Intraoperative recordings of blood flow velocity in aneurysms by means of miniaturized probes (0.2 mm in diameter) with very small sample volume gave no indication of turbulences [69]. The velocities were low and the frequency spectrum showed increased amplitude modulation and signs of increased peripheral flow resistance (Fig. 60).

With the transcranial Doppler sonographic method, blood flow velocities can be registered over the entire diameter of the vessel (0.4 × 0.9 mm). Both the slow flow along the wall and the fast central flow are registered, producing a homogenous frequency distribution in the spectrum.

The transcranial Doppler sonographic examination in more than 90 patients with aneurysms smaller than 1 cm gave no indication of turbulences or any specific changes in the frequency spectrum that would indicate the

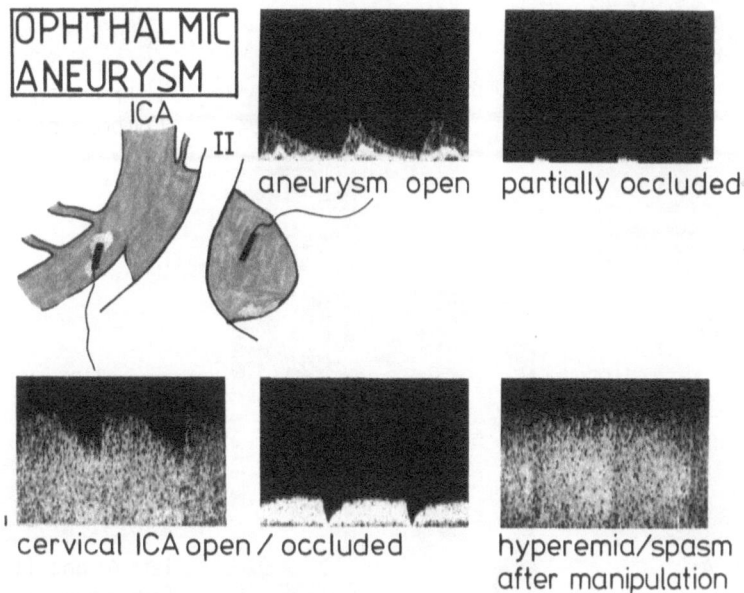

Fig. 60. Intraoperative recordings by high resolution 20 MHz Doppler sonography indicate markedly reduced flow velocity in the aneurysm, no turbulence

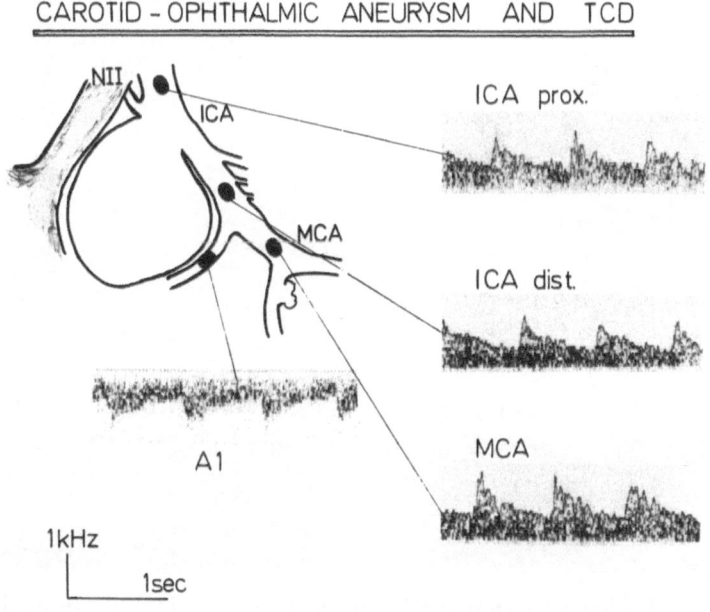

Fig. 61. The flow pattern in the area at the base of a large carotid ophthalmic aneurysm shows no abnormalities. No signs of turbulence or decreased velocity

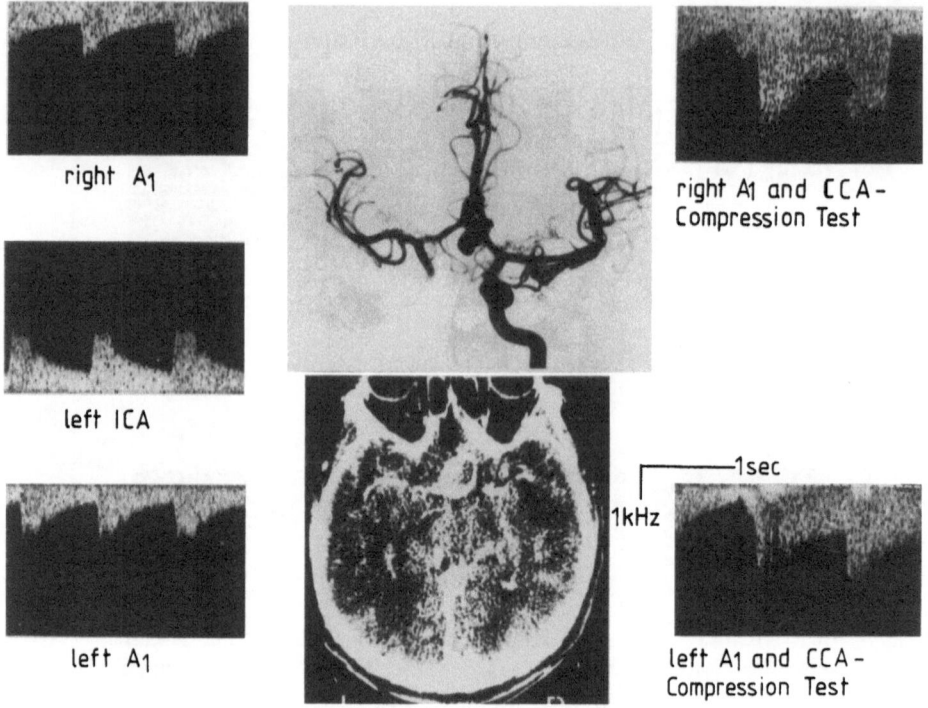

right A₁

left ICA

left A₁

right A₁ and CCA-
Compression Test

—1sec

1kHz

left A₁ and CCA-
Compression Test

Fig. 62. Partially thrombosed ACoA aneurysm. Normal flow pattern in both precommunicating segments of the anterior cerebral arteries, even under compression

GIANT CAROTID BIFURCATION ANEURYSM

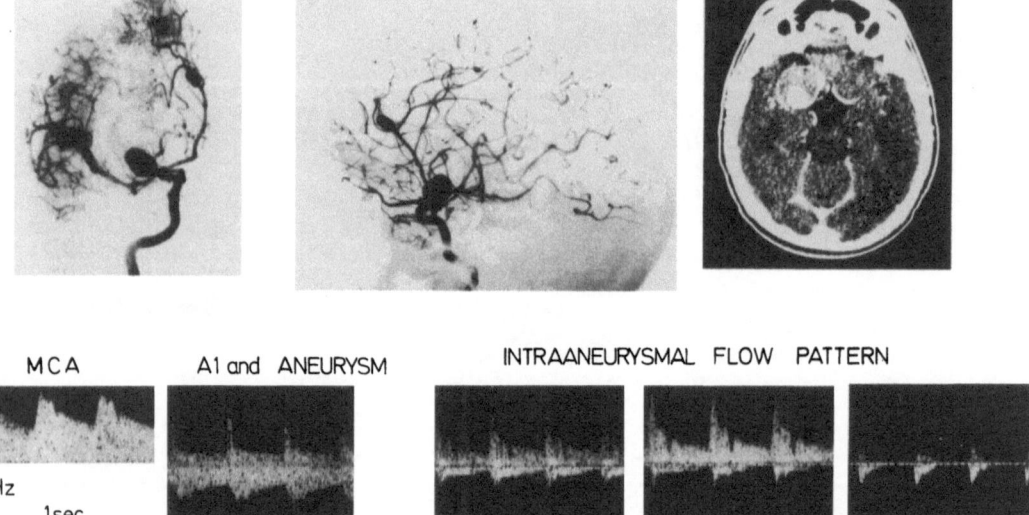

MCA

A1 and ANEURYSM

INTRAANEURYSMAL FLOW PATTERN

1kHz

1sec

Fig. 63. Flow pattern in the feeding arteries of a giant, partially thrombosed carotid bifurcation aneurysm. Normal flow velocity in the MCA. Simultaneous registration of Doppler shifts from the right A1 and one part of the aneurysm. There are sharp systolic peaks and low diastolic velocities indicating high resistance in the aneurysm. The aneurysmal flow pattern shows the same very low frequencies and multi-systolic peak frequencies, no turbulence

presence of an aneurysm (Figs. 61 and 62). If, however, the size of the aneurysm is almost the same as the sample volume in the transcranial Doppler sonographic examination, frequency spectra typical for aneurysm can be recorded: low flow velocities, signs of increased peripheral flow resistance, many low frequencies (bruits) (Figs. 63 and 64). In three patients we found multi-peaked systolic recordings in the frequency spectrum.

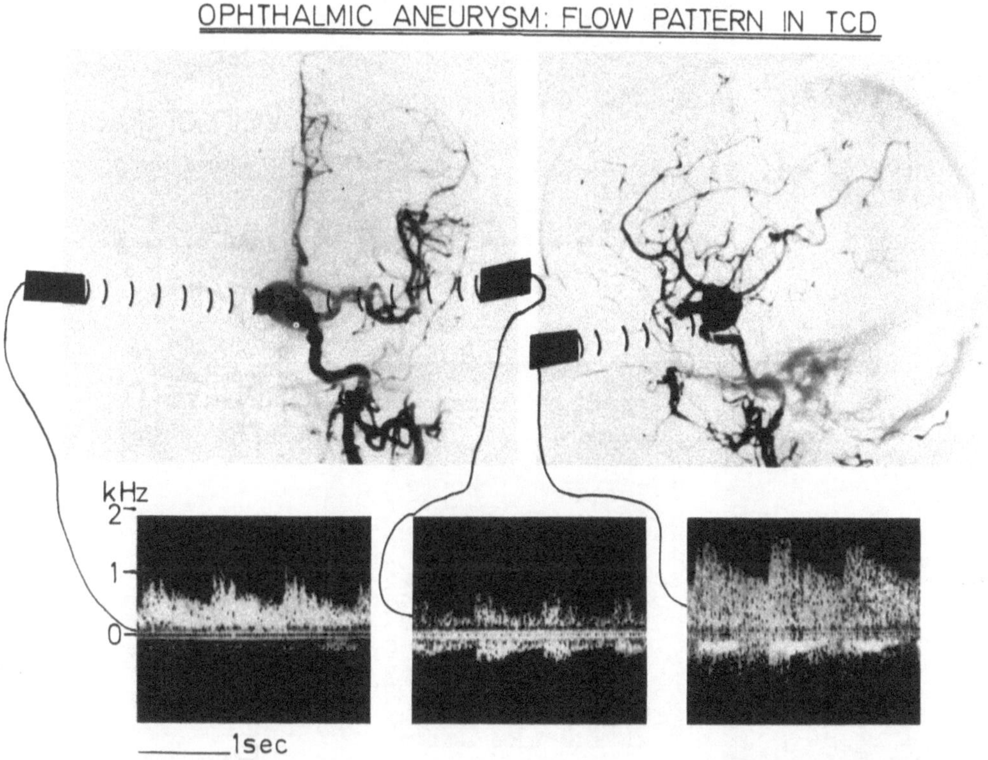

Fig. 64. With the aneurysm flow pattern, transcranial Doppler examination shows very low Doppler shifts and three velocity peaks in the systole, which are typical signs of an intra-aneurysmal flow pattern

Since intraoperative Doppler sonography gives no indication of turbulences in the blood flow in aneurysms, no typical Doppler signals are to be expected in the transcranial Doppler sonographic recordings of aneurysms smaller than 1 cm in diameter. In larger aneurysms, increased energy at the lower frequencies is found. The multiple frequency peaks registered in systole might correspond to the different blood layers that have laminar flow but different velocities.

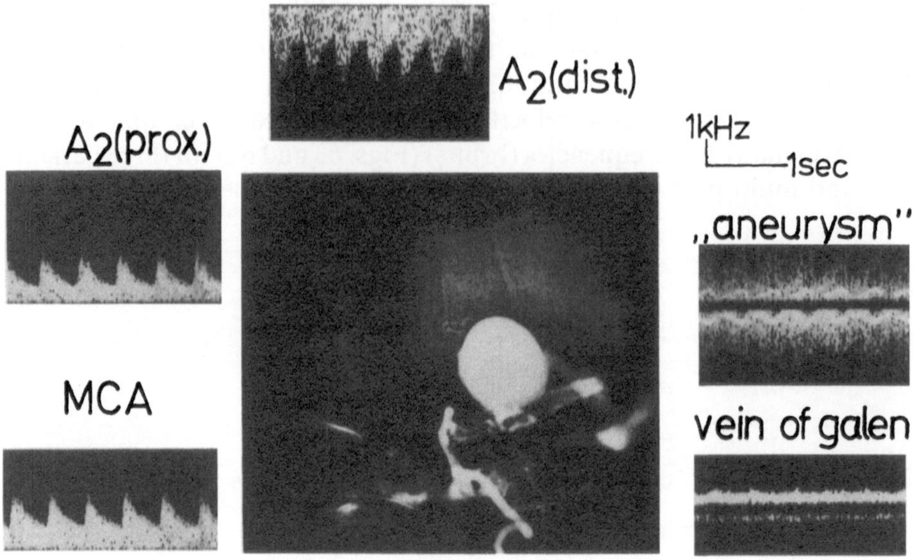

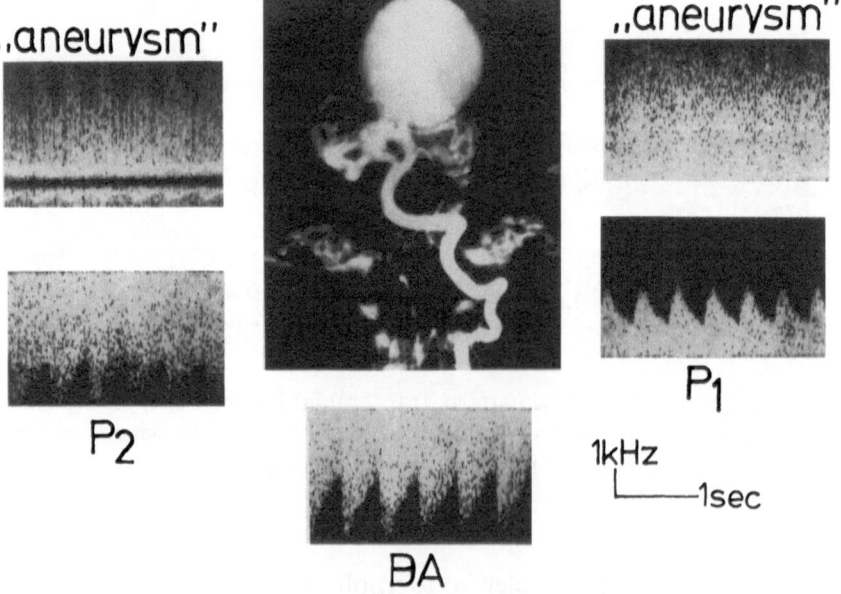

A_2(prox.)

A_2(dist.)

1kHz
1sec

"aneurysm"

MCA

vein of galen

Fig. 65

"aneurysm"

"aneurysm"

P_2

P_1

BA

1kHz
1sec

Fig. 66

Figs. 65 and 66. Two-month old baby with arteriovenous malformation of the vein of Galen. Normal blood flow velocity in the MCA and A 2. Marked velocity increase inside the aneurysm with musical murmurs. Marked velocity increase in the basilar artery and in the right P 2 segment of the posterior cerebral artery as a result of the large arterial venous fistula with very low vascular resistance

Special Case: Vein of Galen—AVM

In the case of an aneurysm of the vein of Galen there is a very high pressure gradient between the arterial and venous segments. The perfusion pressure is thus very high and high velocities are measured transcranially (Figs. 65 and 66) in the aneurysm.

Musical murmurs on both sides of the zero line, broadened frequency spectra, and high diastolic flow velocities can be identified. The hemodynamics of these aneurysms behaves much differently than that of "normal" aneurysms. Aneurysms of the vein of Galen show a very low flow resistance with resulting high intra-aneurysmal blood flow velocities, while normal aneurysms have a high flow resistance and low flow velocities.

Extracranial-intracranial Bypass

Introduction

Intraoperative hemodynamic studies on bypass operations have been carried out using electromagnetic flow measurements [42, 196] fluorescein angiography [120], and Doppler sonography [39, 63, 69, 77, 139]. The patency of the anastomosis has been established postoperatively by the Doppler method [69, 76, 77, 83, 89, 193], by rCBF measurements [73, 199] or by angiography.

Angiography shows the direction of flow in the cerebral arteries and the anatomy of the arteries. The disadvantages of the method however, are that it provides only indirect information on the hemodynamics and it can only be carried out once or twice.

Transcranial Doppler sonography makes it possible to investigate the intracranial hemodynamics before and after surgery. The flow velocities in the middle cerebral artery and in the circle of Willis in patients with occlusion of the internal carotid artery can be followed before and after an extracranial-intracranial bypass operation. Compression tests must be carried out to test the contribution of the bypass to the circulation in the brain.

Method

Using transcranial Doppler sonography we investigated the intracranial blood flow velocities in the major cerebral arteries in patients with occlusion of one or more of the brain-supplying arteries. In cases of occlusive disease, it is particulary important to investigate the collateral pathways: the flow direction and velocity in the precommunicating segment of the anterior cerebral artery (A 1) and the flow velocities in the posterior cerebral artery or basilar artery. The flow patterns in both MCAs are also important because they may represent the hemodynamic effect in the terminal vascular bed of an occlusive disease. The perioperative Doppler ultrasonic examination procedure is shown in Table 11.

Before and after the operation, the systolic, diastolic, and timed-averaged peak frequencies were estimated for each identified vessel. After

Table 11. Perioperative Doppler ultrasonic examination procedure in patients undergoing extracranial-intracranial bypass surgery

Investigated vessel	Information/reason for the investigation
A) Preoperative	
Middle cerebral artery (right and left)	Systolic and diastolic flow velocities, difference in side, damped wave forms?
Precommunicating segment of anterior cerebral artery	Retrograde flow direction? Increased velocity due to collateral flow
Posterior cerebral artery and basilar artery	Increased flow velocity due to collateral flow
B) Postoperative	
Superficial temporal artery	Patency, flow direction
Recipient vessel distally and proximally	Flow direction, flow change reaction to STA-compression
Anterior cerebral artery posterior cerebral artery and basilar artery	Change in flow or flow direction, change in velocity without and with compression of STA

Perioperative Doppler ultrasonic examination procedure in patients undergoing extracranial-intracranial bypass surgery.

the bypass operation, recordings of the trunk and the distal segments of the MCA were carried out with and without compression of the STA. Aditionally, the change in flow direction of the anastomosed branch of the MCA and in the A1 were registered.

Patients

In 10 patients with occlusion of one internal carotid artery, the flow pattern in both MCAs and A1 or P1 could be investigated before and after the operation. Postoperative STA compression tests were performed in 10 patients with unilateral ICA occlusion, in five patients with bilateral ICA occlusion, and in two patients with an ICA cervically occluded with a Salibi clamp for treatment of a cavernous aneurysm. One patient with an occlusion of the vertebral artery was treated with a PICA bypass and two patients with giant fusiform, partially thrombosed MCA aneurysms were treated by bypass only.

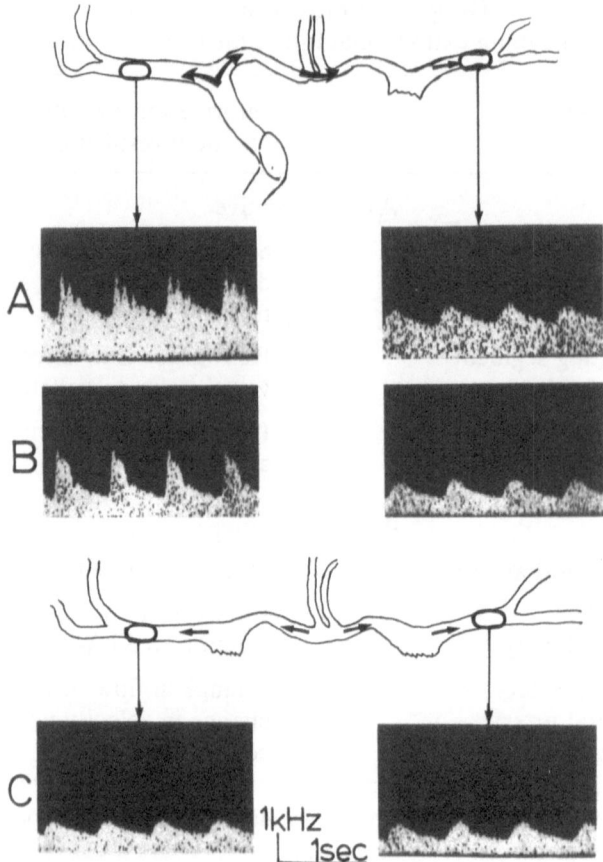

Fig. 67. Damped waveforms in the frequency spectra of the MCA in 2 patients with occlusion of one ICA (*A* and *B*). The patient B had occlusion of both internal carotid arteries and damped waveforms in both MCAs

Results

In about 10% of the patients with occlusive disease, the thickness of the skull made it impossible to obtain reliable recordings. All of the symptomatic patients who were operated on showed lower velocities in the MCA on the side of the ICA occlusion than, on the other side, or they had normal values. In the spectogram the systolic peak was broadenend and the amplitude reduced (damped waveforms) (Fig. 67). In two patients with asymptomatic ICA occlusion, the flow patterns in both MCAs were regular due to a sufficient collateral flow (Fig. 68). In these cases, we did not see any indication for bypass operation.

ASYMPTOMATIC CERVICAL INTERNAL CAROTID OCCLUSION

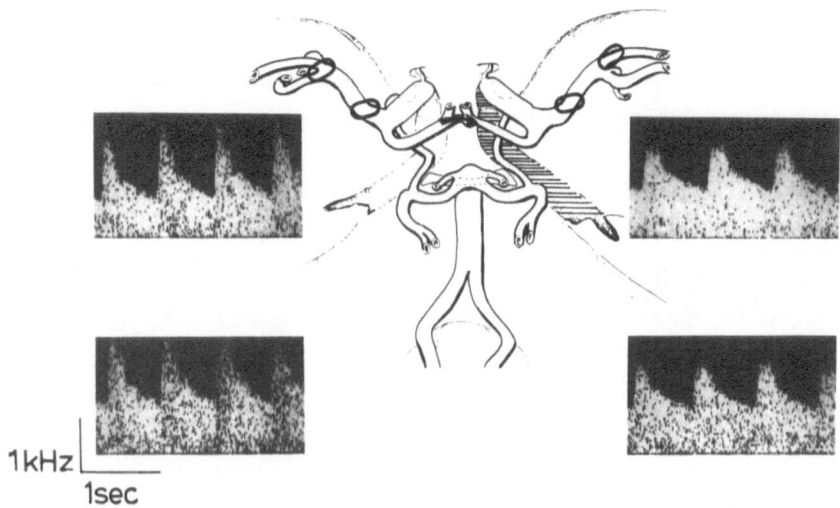

Fig. 68. Occlusion of the right carotid artery. Normal flow pattern in both MCAs

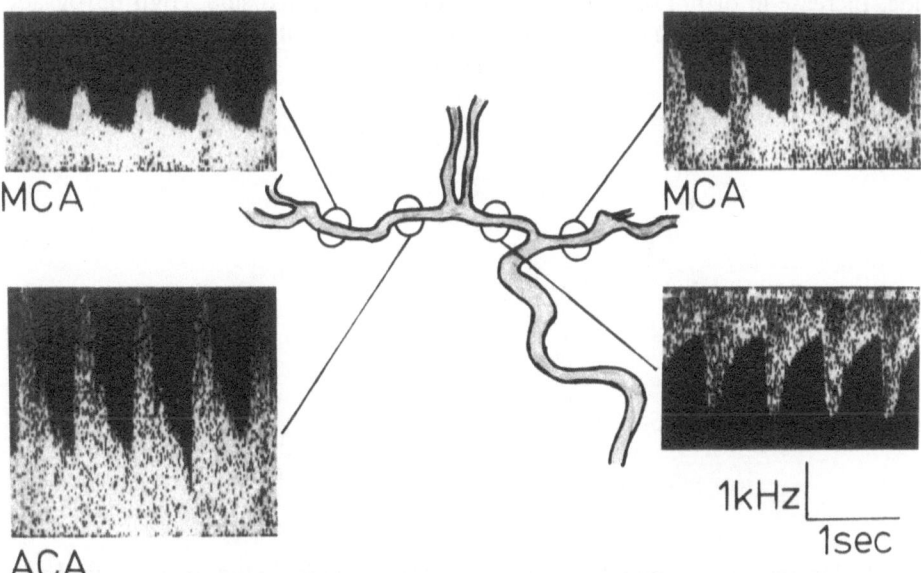

Fig. 69. Occlusion of the left carotid artery. Only slightly damped waveforms in the left MCA due to good collateral flow through the anterior communicating artery

The precommunicating segment of the anterior cerebral artery (A1) of the occluded side showed retrograde flow direction in each case. These findings corresponded well with the results of angiography (Fig. 69).

According to the findings of intraoperative Doppler investigations, postoperatively there must be a retrograde flow with a high velocity in at

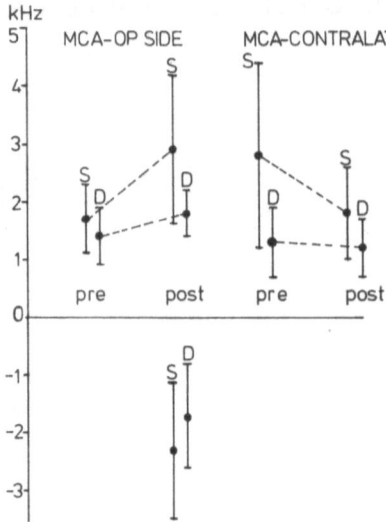

Fig. 70. Mean and standard deviation of the systolic (S) and diastolic (D) flow velocities in the MCA on the side of the bypass operation and on the contralateral side. Increase in orthograde flow velocity on the operated side. High retrograde flow in one MCA branch on the operated side. Decrease of systolic flow velocity on the contralateral MCA

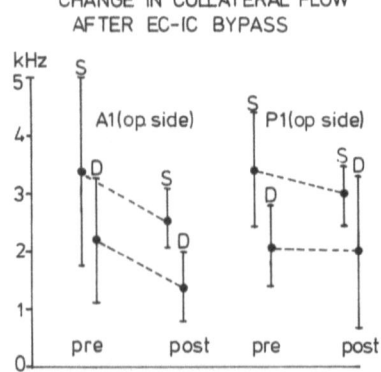

Fig. 71. Decrease of systolic (S) and diastolic (D) velocities in the collateral pathway of A-1 and P-1 after bypass surgery

least one main branch of the MCA to which the bypass is connected. The orthograde flow in the other MCA branches in eight patients showed an increase in the flow velocities as compared with the preoperative findings. The best recordings of the retrograde flow could be obtained at a depth of 3.5 to 4 cm (Fig. 70).

   The flow direction in the A1 did not change after bypass surgery, which means that the original collateral pathway was still used. The velocity in the A1 of the operated side decreased after extracranial-intracranial bypass surgery. In four patients, the preoperative collateral flow came mainly from the P1 segment. Postoperatively, the systolic velocity decreased in this artery (Fig. 71).

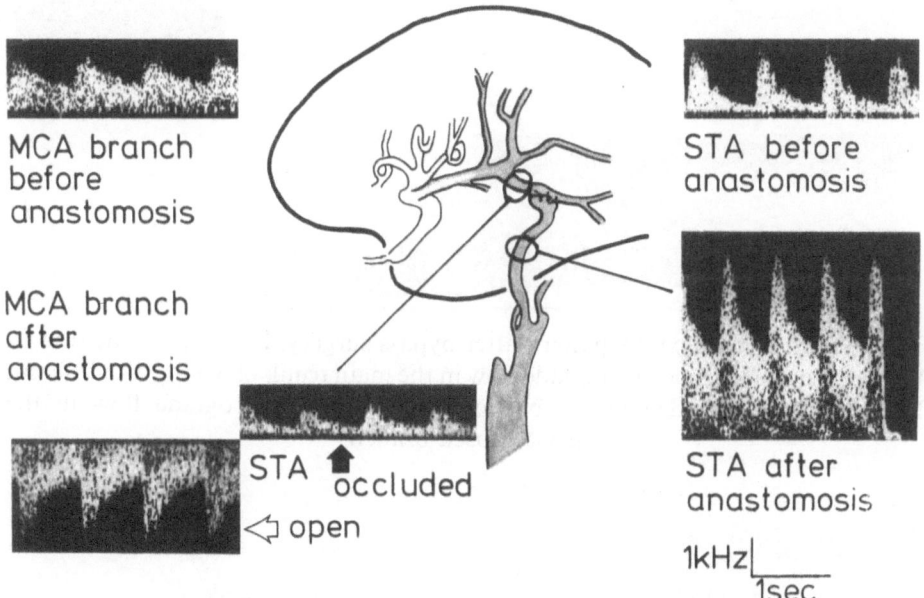

MCA branch
before
anastomosis

MCA branch
after
anastomosis

STA ⬆ occluded
◁ open

STA before
anastomosis

STA after
anastomosis

1kHz⌊___
          1sec

Fig. 72. Bilateral cervical carotid artery occlusion. Low blood flow velocities are damped waveform in the area of the middle cerebral artery. After the extracranial-intracranial bypass procedure, increased velocities and retrograde flow could be observed in the recipient cerebral area, as well as an increase in flow velocity in the donor artery

Results: STA Compression Tests and TCD

After compression of the STA, the orthograde flow velocities in the 19 patients investigated showed the following reactions: the flow velocities remained unchanged in 3 cases; they decreased in eight cases; the velocities dropped to zero in four cases; and, surprisingly, they increased in four cases.

   Representative examples of the change in blood flow velocity and flow direction are given in Figs. 72, 73, and 74. the retrograde flow in one MCA branch induced by the bypass ceased in all of the patients after compression of the STA. When two MCA branches with different flow directions were simultaneously recorded, the orthograde flow was reduced and the retrograde flow ceased.

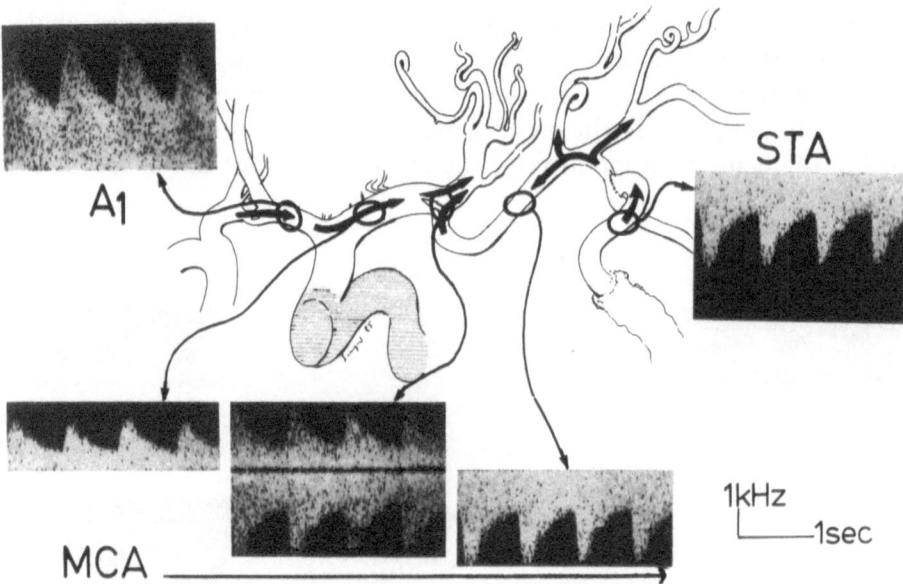

Fig. 73. Hemodynamic flow pattern after bypass surgery: high retrograde flow in A 1 on the occluded side, orthograde flow in the main trunk of MCA, two different flow directions recorded in the bifurcation of MCA, retrograde flow in the anastomosed branch

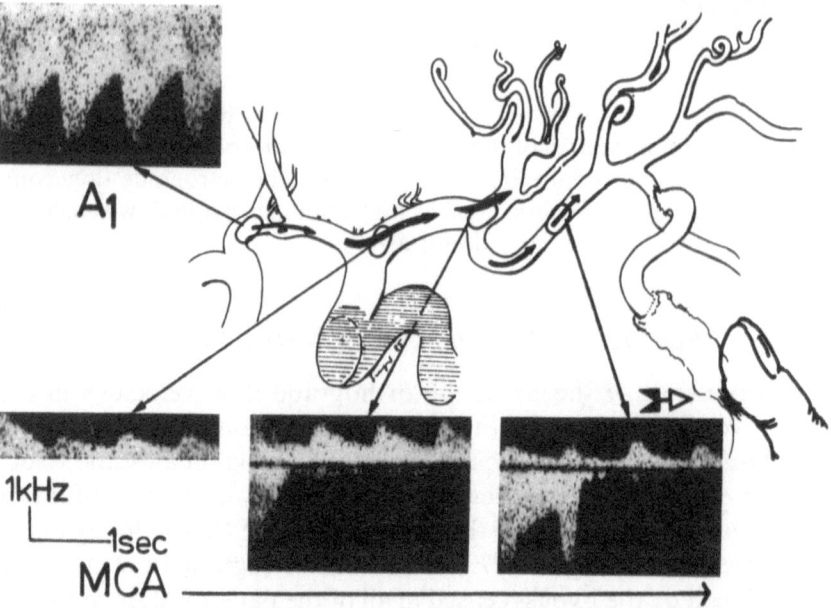

Fig. 74. After compression of the STA the orthograde flow in the MCA trunk is reduced. The retrograde flow stops in the anastomosed MCA branch and the velocities in the MCA without orthograde flow are reduced

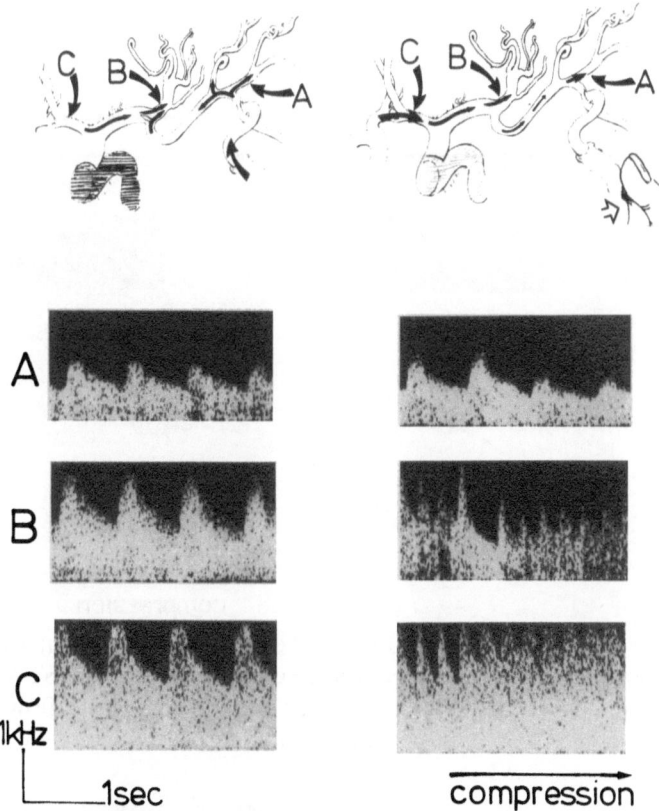

Fig. 75. *A* and *B* Reduction of orthograde flow in MCA after STA compression tests. *C* Increase of collateral flow in A1 on the occluded side due to reduction of perfusion pressure

In four patients we were able to investigate the effect of the bypass on the flow velocity of the A1 collateral (Figs. 75 and 76). In these cases, the velocity in the A1 and MCA increased considerably during compression of the STA as a result of the increased perfusion pressure, which was caused by a decrease of the MCA resistance.

Results: Special Cases

With Doppler sonography, even complex hemodynamic changes in the circle of Willis can be detected (Fig. 77). In a patient with bilateral carotid artery occlusion and unilateral vertebral artery occlusion who underwent bypass surgery on the right side, the blood flow velocity and the collateral supply via A1 and P1 is the same as before surgery, although the bypass function is shown to be very good.

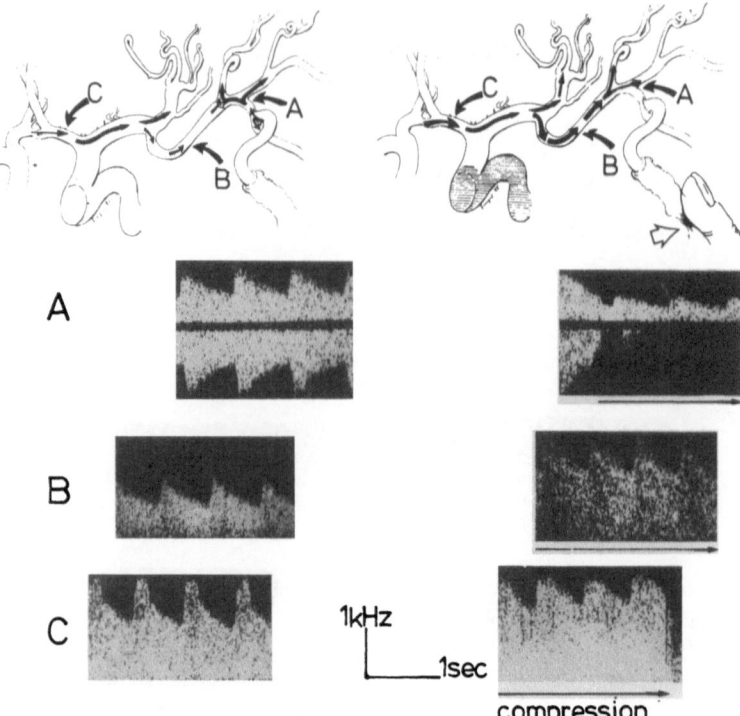

Fig. 76. Increase of flow velocity in A1 (*A*) and even in the main trunk of the MCA (*B*) due to reduced vascular resistance during compression of the STA. Near the anastomosis the retrograde flow direction stops and the orthograde flow is reduced after compression

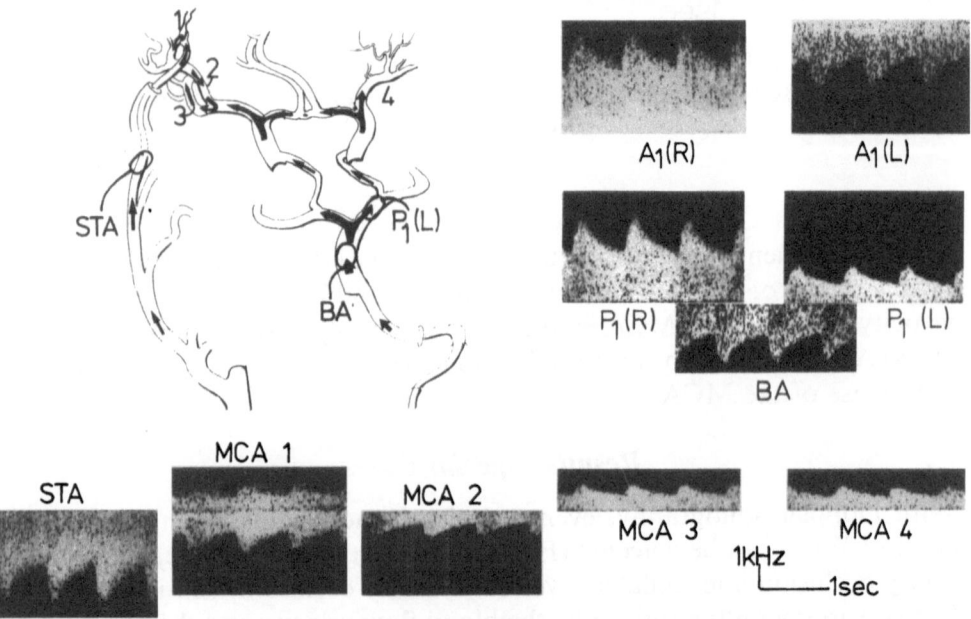

Fig. 77. This patient had an occlusion of both internal carotid arteries in the neck and of the right vertebral artery. After extracanial-intracranial bypass operation on the right side, no change in the frequency spectra in either MCA, continued retrograde flow in A-1 on the right side, and good collateral flow velocity in the basilar artery and the right posterior cerebral artery

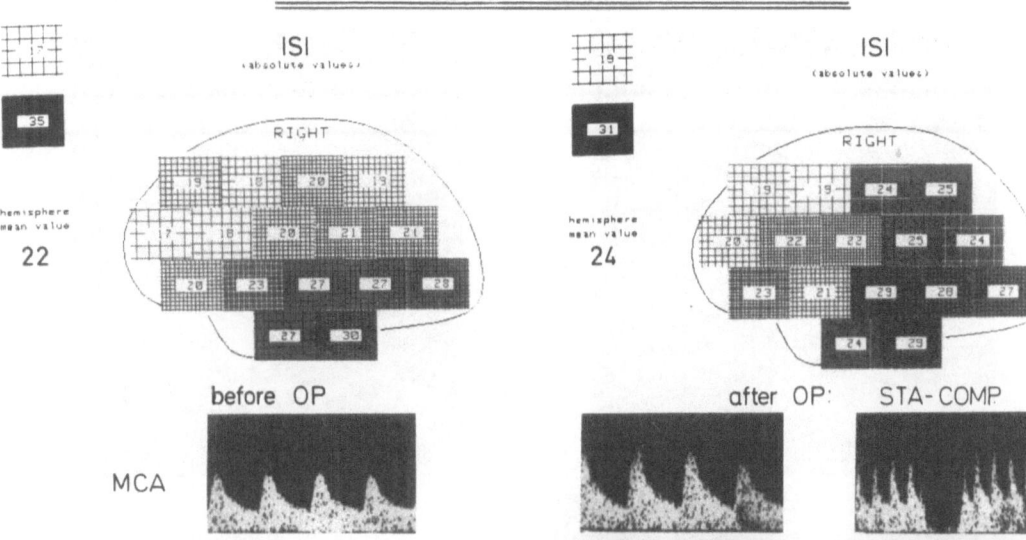

Fig. 78. The cerebral blood flow measurements with the inhalation of xenon compared with the blood flow capacity before and after bypass operation: there is no significant change in either the cerebral blood flow or in the velocity and the frequency spectra. (The author is very indebted to Prof. Dr. G. Meinig, Dept. of Neurosurgery, University of Mainz, Federal Republic of Germany, for giving us the opportunity to carry out this investigation)

Results: Comparison of CBF Measurements with Transcranial Doppler Sonography

The cases shown in Fig. 78 clearly shows reduced blood flow values using the [133]Xenon inhalation technique. After bypass surgery on the right side there is an increase in velocity in the MCA and in the blood flow measurement in the frontal and parieto-occipital areas.

One patient with moya-moya disease and progressive stenosis of the internal carotid artery was followed up with Doppler sonography for 2 ½ years. During this time extracranial-intracranial bypass surgery was carried out on both sides. The clinical symptoms including sensory disturbances, speech and reading disturbances, and focal senso-motor deficits were not improved by the surgery, but the stenosis of the ICA was progressive. After the bypass operation the blood flow velocities measured by transcranial

ICA STENOSIS AND COLLATERAL-FLOW IN MOYA MOYA

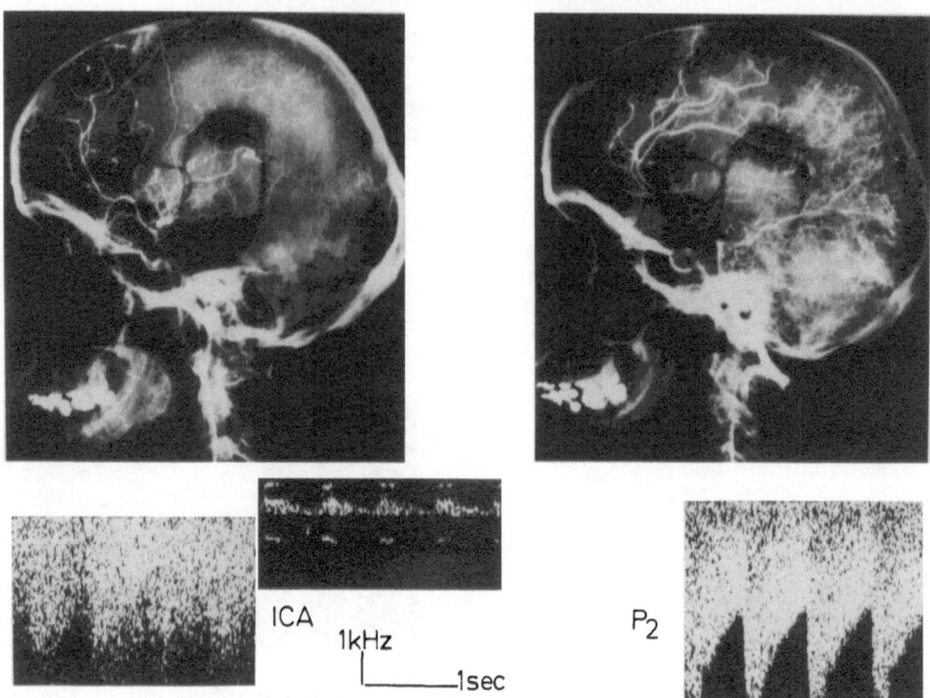

Fig. 79. 29-year-old women suffering from moya-moya disease in both hemispheres with high grade internal carotid artery stenosis. Angiography shows good collateral flow from the posterior cerebral arteries supplying nearly the entire territory of the anterior cerebral artery. Extracranial-intracranial anastomosis had been performed on both sides. There are high velocities in the supraclinoid segment of the carotid artery with musical murmurs, indicating arterial wall vibrations. The blood flow velocity in the posterior cerebral artery increased more than four times the normal value due to high collateral flow

Doppler sonography and by regional CBF measurements were only temporarily improved (Figs. 79 and 80).

Discussion

Doppler ultrasound can demonstrate the patency of an anastomosis by establishing a change from the external type flow pattern in the STA to the internal type and an increase in flow velocity. Hyodo [89] and Müller [144] measured the efficiency of the bypass with the ultrasonic quantitative flow measurement before and during compression of the STA. The measurements were made in the common carotid artery and the decrease of blood

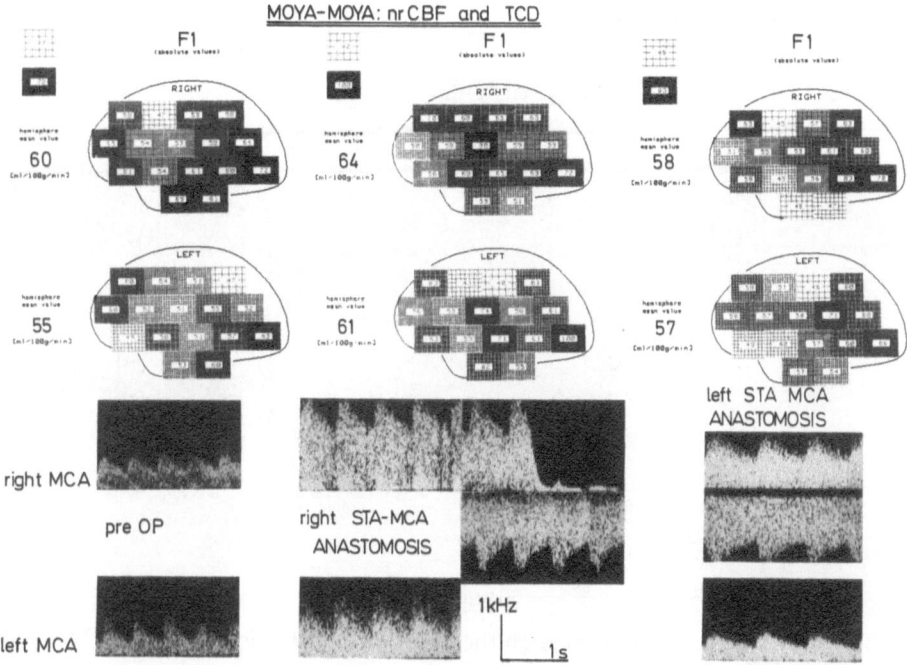

Fig. 80. Cerebral blood flow measurements and transcranial Doppler findings in the patient shown in Fig. 79. After the bypass operation on the right side, the blood flow velocities in both MCAs have increased and the CBF measurements show better perfusion of the brain. Four months later, after extracranial-intracranial anastomosis on the left side had been peformed, the CBF investigation reveals a reduction over the previous findings, even though transcranial Doppler shows good functioning of the anastomosis

flow in the artery showed indirectly to what extent the STA blood flow took part in the brain circulation. Apart from the pure patency, we are now able to measure noninvasively the hemodynamic effect of the bypass circulation in the MCA and in the circle of Willis.

The example in Fig. 81 with normal MCA velocities, good collateral flow, and a marked cerebral infarction in the CT scan shows that the velocity recordings alone do not provide a sufficient basis for the decision to operate. In this cases, the brain infarction was probably the result of an embolism and not of hypoperfusion. In such a case, of course, there is no indication for bypass surgery. Fig. 82 shows, on the other hand, that there are damped waveforms in the left MCA but infarction is revealed by CT, in which case bypass surgery is not indicated. Significantly reduced MCA velocities on the side of the ICA occlusion, however, may be a sign of still asymptomatic low perfusion and preventive bypass surgery may be considered.

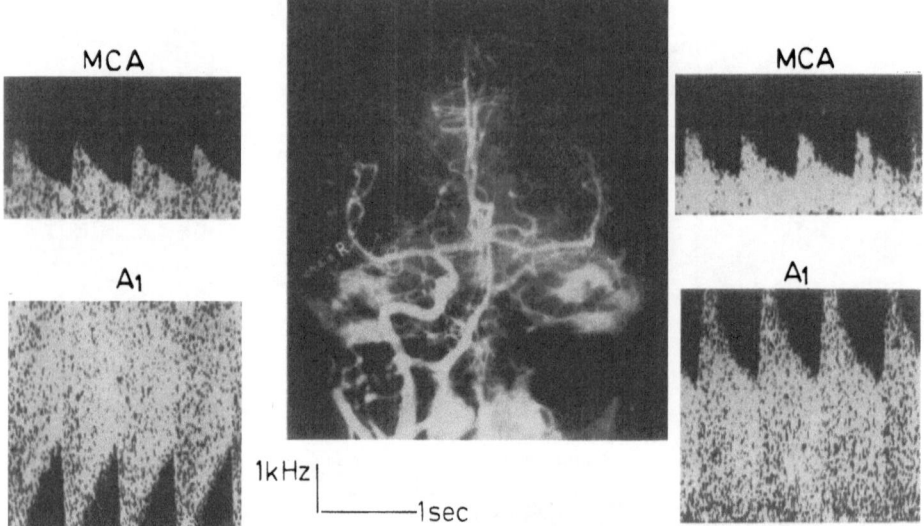

Fig. 81. Good collateral flow through the anterior communicating artery. Normal flow pattern in both MCAs, but clinically the patient had severe hemiparesis. No indication for extracranial-intracranial bypass surgery

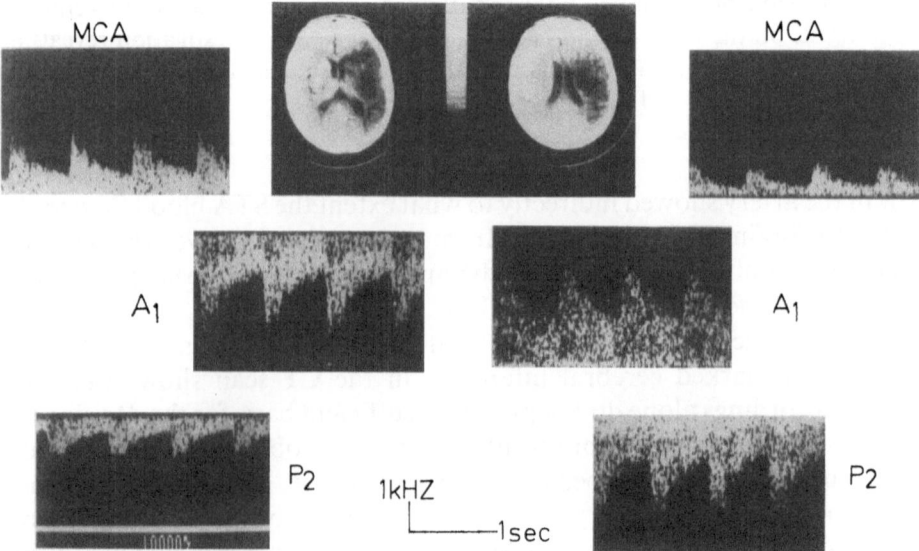

Fig. 82. Marked brain infarction on the left in the CT of a patient with internal carotid artery occlusion on the left side. Damped waveform in MCA on the left side in transcranial Doppler. Collateral flow in the left anterior communicating artery ($A1$) and the left posterior cerebral artery ($P2$). No indication for bypass operation

CERVICAL ICA-STENOSIS   CAROTID ENDARTERECTOMY

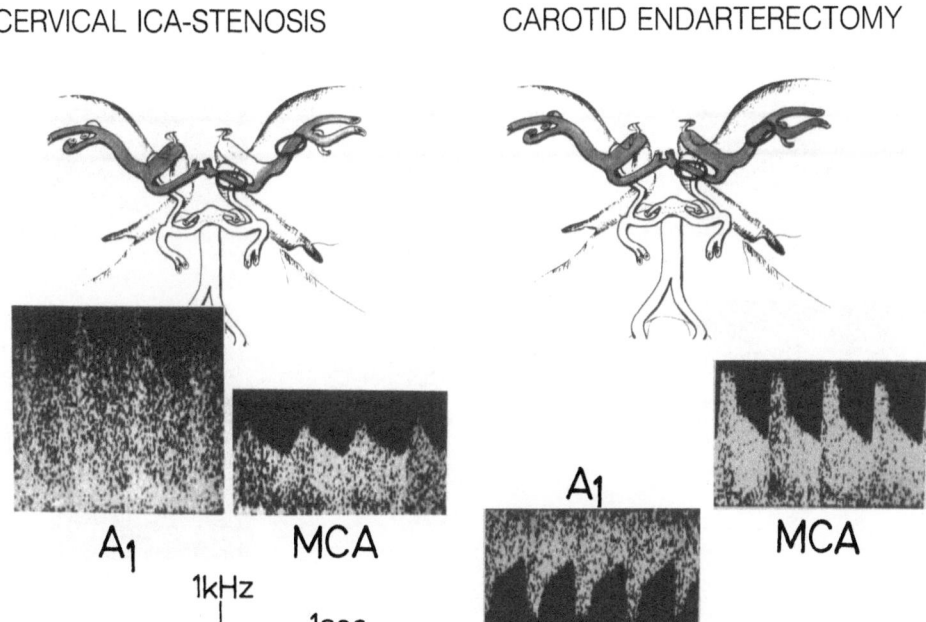

Fig. 83. A patient with stenosis of the cervical internal carotid artery with damped waveforms in MCA and high collateral flow in the precommunicating segment of the anterior cerebral artery. After cervical endarteriectomy, normal flow pattern and flow direction indicating good operative hemodynamic result

Further experience will show whether patients with markedly reduced blood flow velocities in the MCA are at a higher risk of developing ischemic deficits. The retrograde flow in the A1, unlike that following cervical endarterectomy (Fig. 83), did not change after bypass operation.

Austin [14] reported that in cerebral blood flow measurements, not only the affected side, but also the opposite side show reduced perfusion. Postoperatively, the increase in blood flow was 23% on the occluded side and 14% on the opposite side. He attributed this to an intracerebral steal by a cross-over via the anterior communicating artery and posterior communicating artery. The same phenomenon can be confirmed by our transcranial Doppler findings: postoperative reduction of A1 collateral flow and an increase in the A1 by compression of the STA. When discussing Doppler results, one must always bear in mind that the blood flow is mainly dependent on the blood pressure, the width of the arteries, and the peripheral resistance. The latest results of the international bypass study [21] reveal that among the patients studied, surgery produced no better results than conservative therapy alone. It cannot be established from the method and from the inclusion criterion, however, to what extent the neurological deficits of the patients were caused by ischemia or by

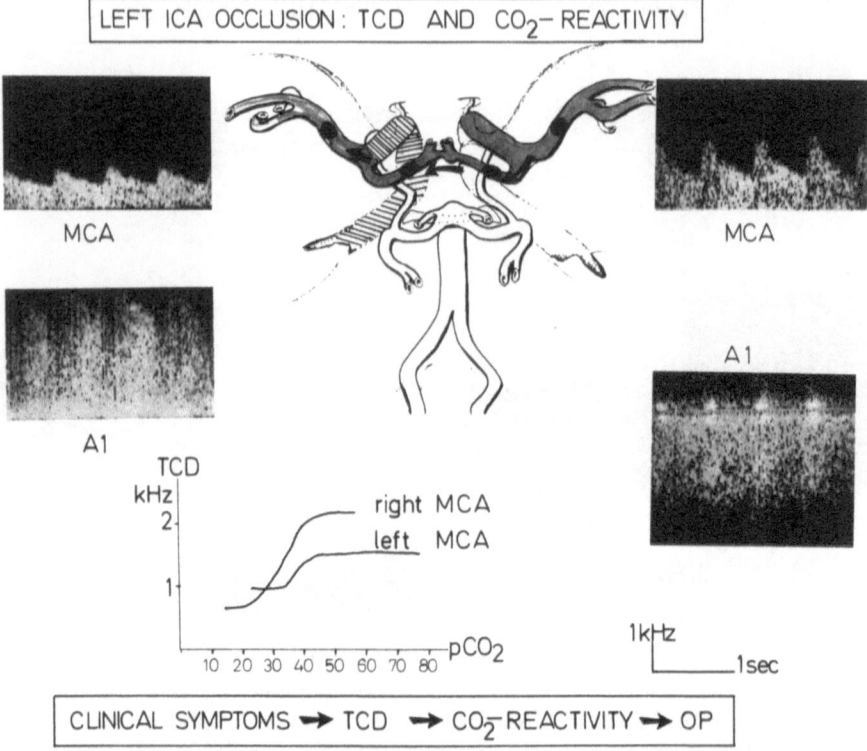

Fig. 84. Patient with internal carotid artery occlusion on the left side. There is good collateral flow from the right to the left side via the anterior communicating artery. The flow pattern in the left MCA shows slightly damped waveforms. The CO_2 reactivity of the diastolic flow velocities in both MCAs is reduced on the left side, which may be an indication for bypass surgery

embolism. To arrive at an objective answer to this question, function tests should be carried out during the transcranial Doppler investigation or during the CBF measurements (Figs. 84 and 85).

In transcranial Doppler sonography, a well-functioning bypass is indicated by a high retrograde flow in one branch of the MCA, a higher orthograde flow than before surgery, and a bidirectional flow in the region of the anastomosis. The compensatory retrograde direction of flow in the A1 on the occluded side is not altered by the bypass. In a well-functioning bypass, which means that there is a high pressure gradient between the donor and recipient arteries, the natural collateral circulation is diminished. In these cases the blood flow velocity in the main branch of the MCA is reduced, which can result in reduced perfusion in the region supplied by the lenticulostriate arteries.

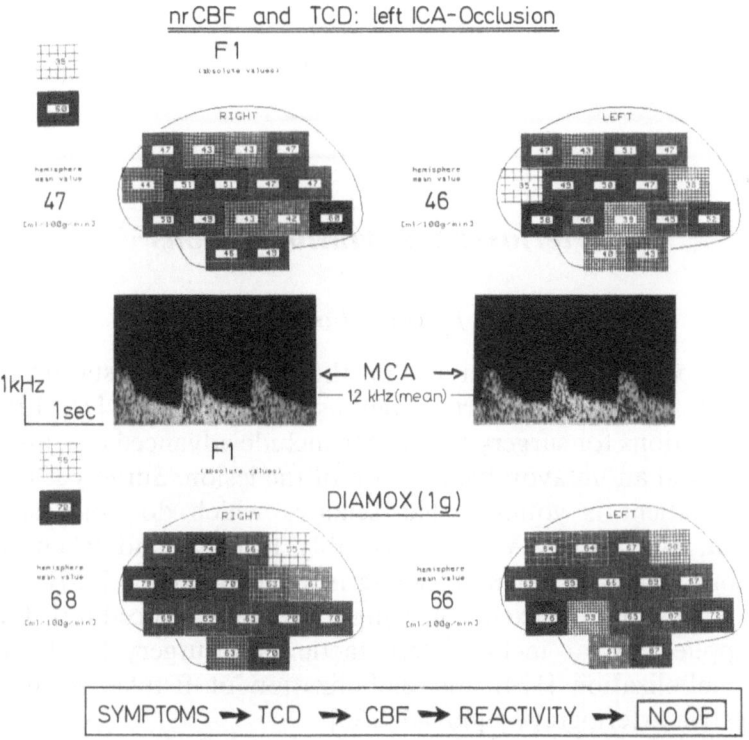

Fig. 85. Occlusion of the left internal carotid artery resulted in a moderate reduction of cerebral blood flow in both hemispheres. The transcranial Doppler measurements show slightly reduced frequencies in both MCAs. Application of diamox results in good reactivity, which is shown in the CBF measurements. There is no indication for bypass operation

Arteriovenous Malformations

Introduction

There have been numerous studies on the clinical manifestation and the natural history of cerebral arteriovenous malformations [71, 125, 159]. Contraindications for surgery for AVMs include advanced age, absence of symptoms, and an unfavorable location of the lesion. Surgery is indicated when the patient is younger, has seizures which do not respond to medication, when the AVM is favorably located, and when there is intracerebral space-occupying bleeding from the angioma [157].

Apart from surgical exclusion (single or staged procedure), the techniques applied so far include stereotactic radiosurgery [195], artificial surgical embolization [124] and embolization of fistulas by means of superselective arteriography [46, 47, 135].

Despite the employment of refined microsurgical techniques for angioma surgery [152, 181–183, 212], the hemodynamic conversion of shunt flow to perfusion flow is responsible for the still unsolved problem of postoperative complications such as cerebral edema and diffuse intracerebral hemorrhage near the operative area or other locations.

Hemodynamic changes have been described on the basis of cerebral blood flow measurements (CBF), fluorescein angiography, intraoperative Doppler sonography, and electromagnetic blood volume flow measurements [56, 152–155, 202, 209]. In 1978, Spetzler explained the "normal perfusion pressure breakthrough theory". According to this theory, "when normal perfusion was suddenly re-established following resection of the AVM, the chronically ischemic hemisphere might not be able to regulate this new pressure, leading to capillary breakthrough resulting in edema and, if severe enough, hemorrhage".

The transcranial Doppler sonographic examination method now makes it possible to study the influence of arteriovenous shunts in cerebral angiomas on the blood flow velocity in the circle of Willis and in the proximal MCA. Several examples are presented illustrating these changes before and after surgical exclusion and superselective embolization *.

---

* The author is greatly indepted to Professor J. J. Merland (Paris), who allowed him to carry out transcranial Doppler recordings on patients in his department.

AVM HEMODYNAMICS : ANGIOGRAPHY AND TCD

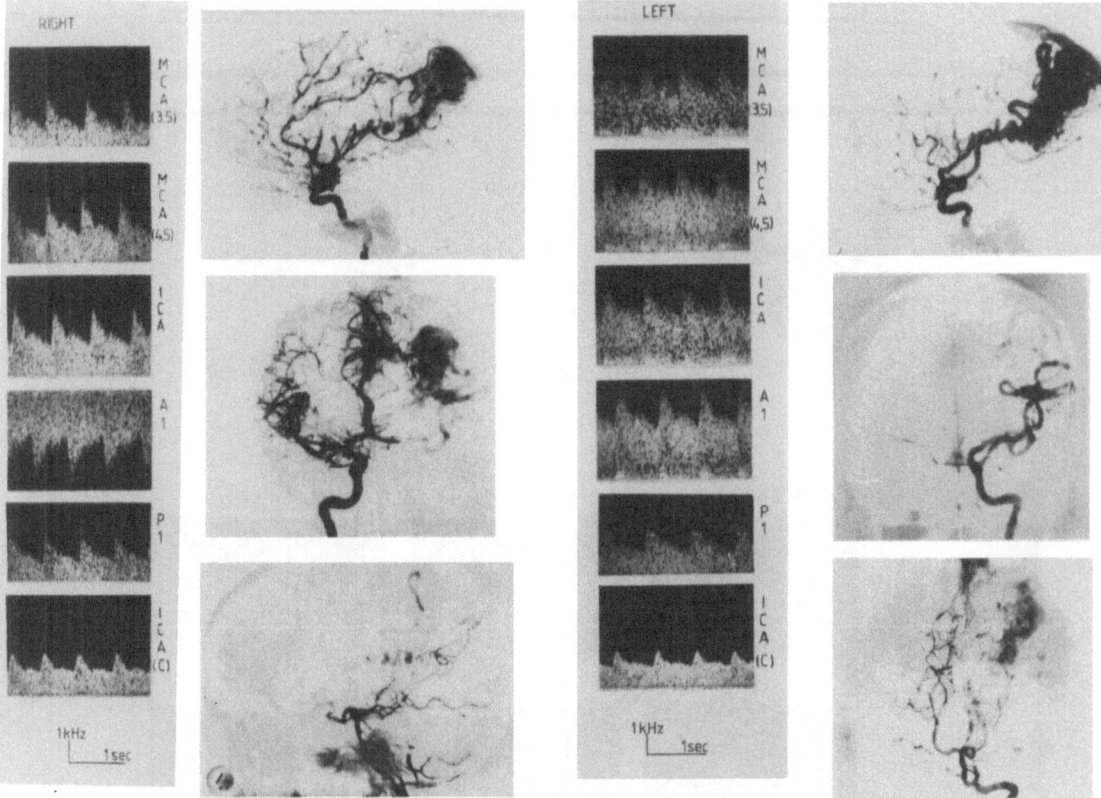

Fig. 86. Increased velocities up to 3 kHz in diastole in the feeding arteries (MCA, ICA, and A1 on both sides). The hemodynamic steal effect in angiography corresponds to a retrograde flow direction in the right A1. Frequency spectra in MCA and ICA on the right side are normal

Transcranial Doppler investigations were carried out in 11 patients before and after surgery. Measurements could be made in six patients before and after superselective embolization and five patients were examined without surgery.

The question to be addressed is whether the transcranial Doppler investigation method enables arteriovenous malformations to be classified according to hemodynamic aspects in order to prevent postoperative bleeding.

Feeding Arteries and Steal Effect

The high pressure gradient between the feeding arteries and the efferent vessels of an AVM effects an increase in the blood flow velocity in the

AVM AND CO₂-REACTIVITY IN TCD

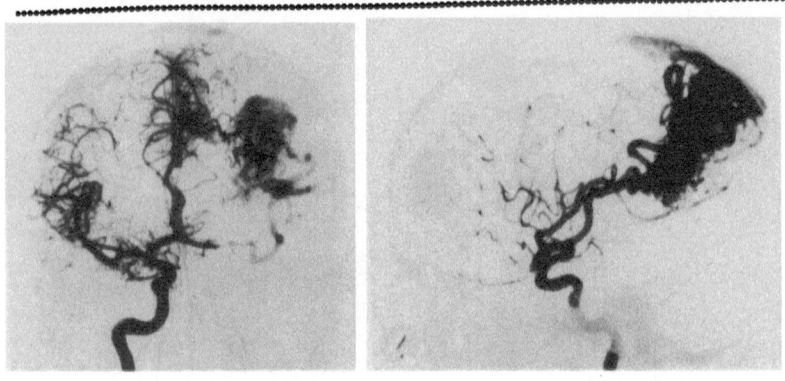

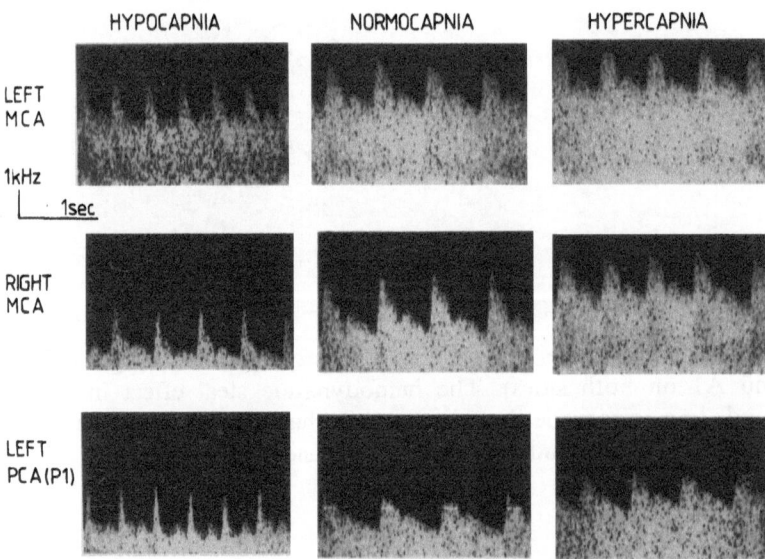

Fig. 87. Reduced CO_2 reactivity in the left MCA—range of diastolic flow velocity 1.4 kHz. The right MCA shows a diastolic velocity range of 2.0 kHz. The CO_2-reactivity on the right side is not impaired and on the left side not exhausted

feeding arteries. This happens because there are no regulating capillaries and, as the vessel widens, the velocity increases. The steal effect of the AVM on the circle of Willis can manifest itself in a reversal of the flow direction in the precommunicating segments of the anterior and posterior cerebral arteries and in a reduction of the blood flow velocity in the arteries of the contralateral hemisphere.

The AVM shown in Figs. 86 and 87 has caused a reversal of the flow direction in the A1 with a marked increase in blood flow velocity. The blood continues to be led into the AVM through the posterior communicating artery via the internal carotid artery and the middle cerebral artery. Hypercapnia up to 70 mm Hg was achieved by adding CO_2 to the inhaled air. Hypocapnia was reached by maximum active hyperventilation. The

AVM and TCD

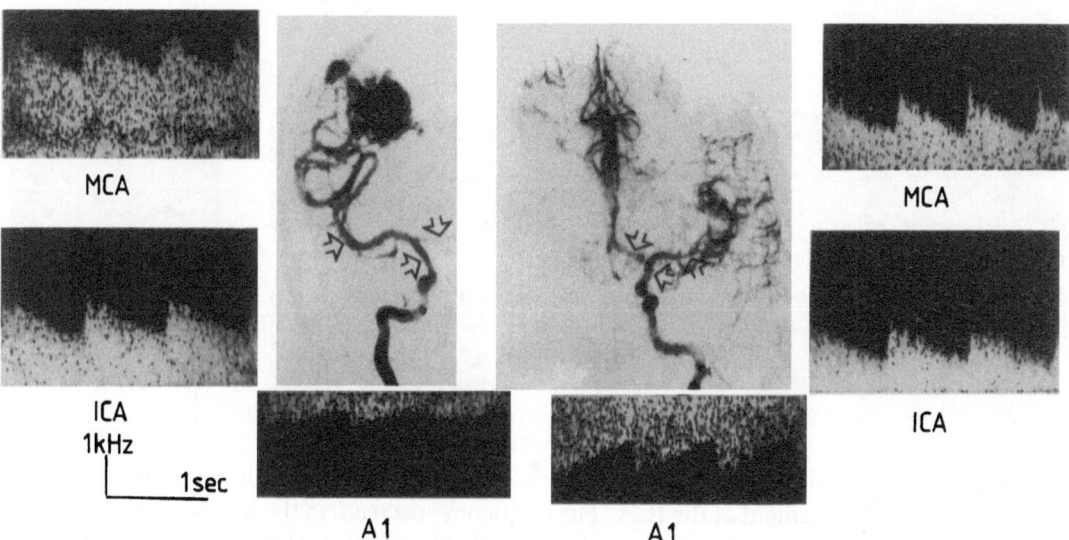

Fig. 88. Steal effect from the angioma resulting in low velocity in the right A1. There is increased velocity in the left A1 because it supplies both pericallosal arteries

brain-supplying vessels were not limited in their CO_2 reactivity, while the feeding arteries showed only slight CO_2 reactivity.

A slight steal effect of the AVM (Fig. 88) can be seen in the A1 on the ipsilateral side, in which there is orthograde flow with reduced velocity. The contralateral A1 supplies both pericallosal arteries, which causes the blood flow velocity to double.

The capacity of the collateral flow can be tested by temporary balloon occlusion during interventional neuroradiology (Fig. 89). This angioma seated in the dominant hemisphere has high velocities in the MCA and in the internal carotid artery. While the contralateral vessels show normal frequency spectra, the velocity in the MCA is considerably reduced by balloon occlusion of the proximal ICA. After distal occlusion of the ICA for 2 minutes, the blood flow velocity through the cortical anastomoses is

TCD AND DIAGNOSTIC OCCLUSION OF ICA AND MCA

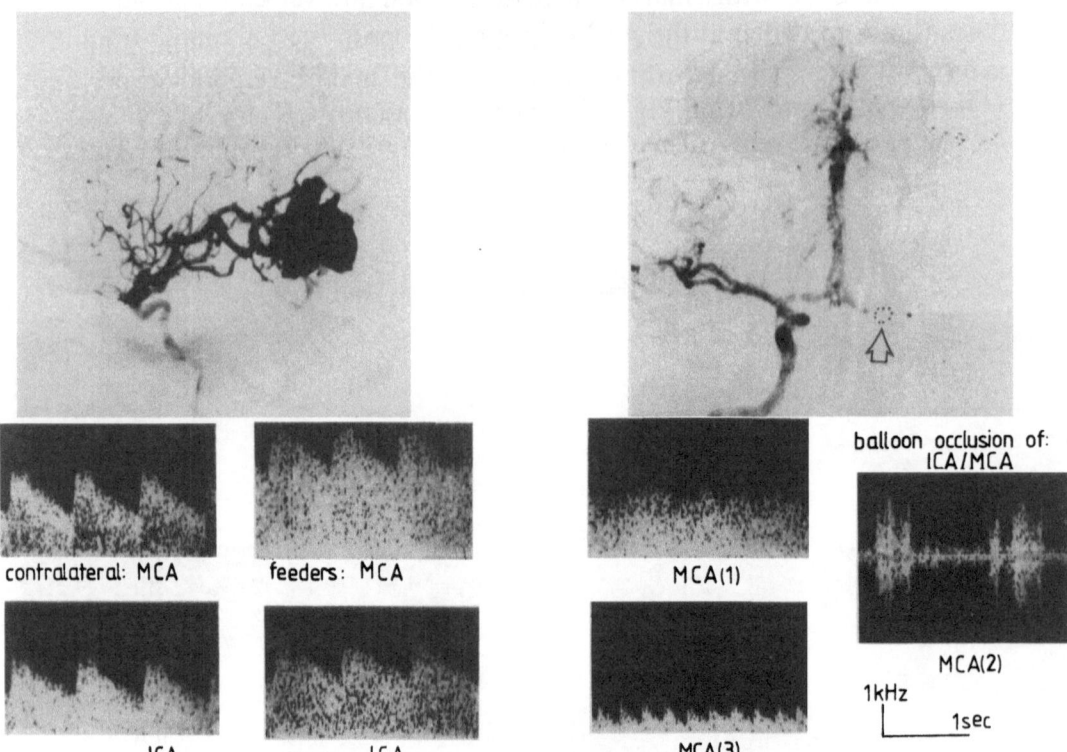

Fig. 89. Collateral flow capacity in the circle of Willis is shown by balloon occlusion of the proximal segment of the ICA. The frequency spectrum in the MCA (*1*) shows reduced velocity with a damped waveform. Balloon occlusion of the main trunk of the MCA shows zero flow during occlusion and increase of flow when the balloon is deflated. Occlusion of the proximal part of the MCA (*3*) results in a delayed onset of reduced flow velocity due to cortical anastomosis

reduced after a brief period of latency. When the MCA is directly occluded, blood flow velocity can no longer be measured by transcranial Doppler sonography.

SAH and AVM

In carrying out transcranial measurement of blood flow velocities, it must be taken into account that angiomas often manifest themselves clinically by spontaneous subarachnoid hemorrhage [159]. Fig. 90 shows the correlation of the frequency spectra with the angiographic findings prior to the SAH.

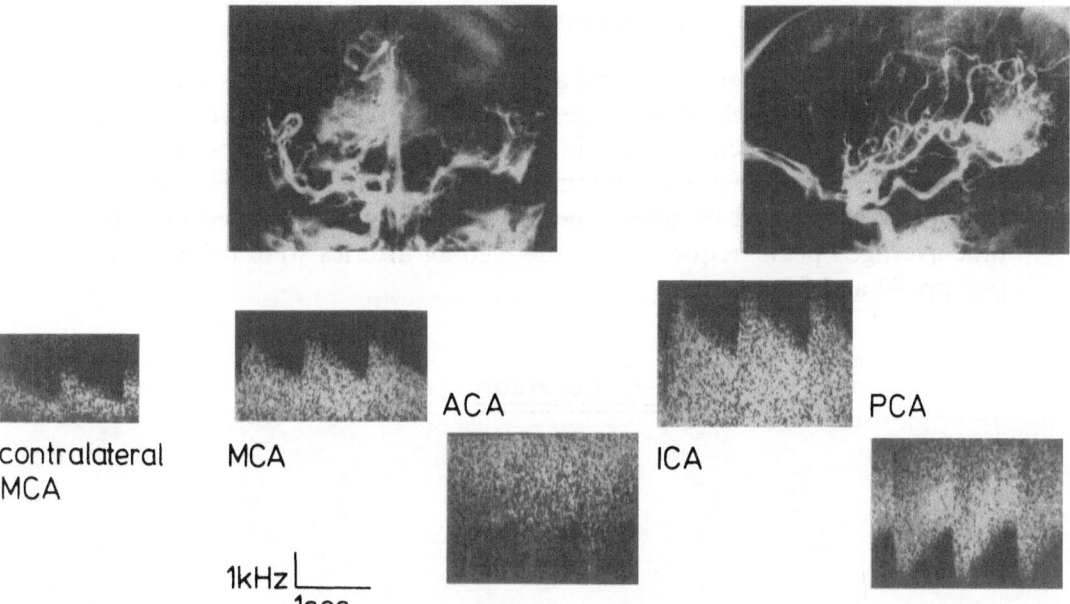

Fig. 90. Increase flow velocity in the feeding arteries. The arteries with the highest velocities have the largest diameter

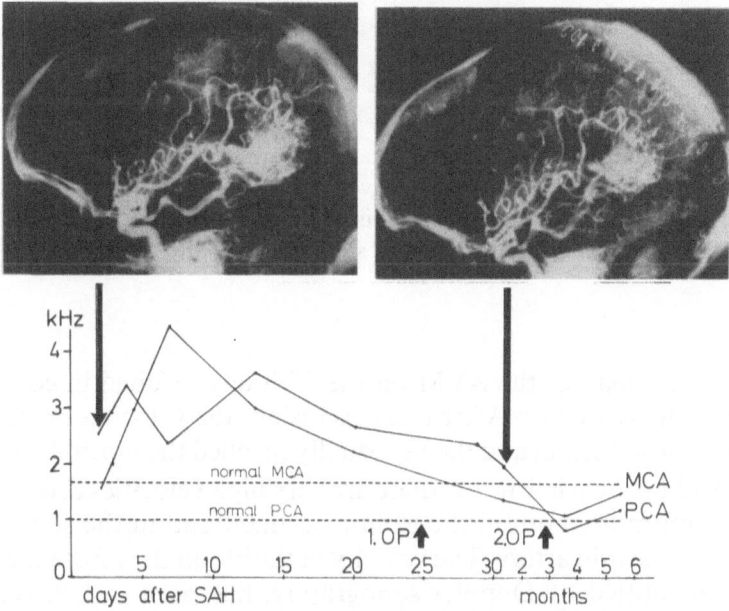

Fig. 91. After SAH from the angioma, the velocities increased in the MCA and PCA in the first 10 days. As a result of vasospasm they then decreased. After the incomplete first occlusion of the AVM, the velocities did not decrease immediately. After total resection they did

The posterior and anterior cerebral arteries have the largest vessel diameter
with the highest Doppler frequencies, while the MCA has a lower velocity.
Fig. 91 shows the velocity changes in the MCA and in the posterior cerebral
artery in the same patients during the first 25 days after SAH. The changes
in velocity are caused by SAH, and AVM surgery was delayed until the
time-averaged peak frequencies in the feeding arteries were below 3 kHz
(see pp. 70 and 71).

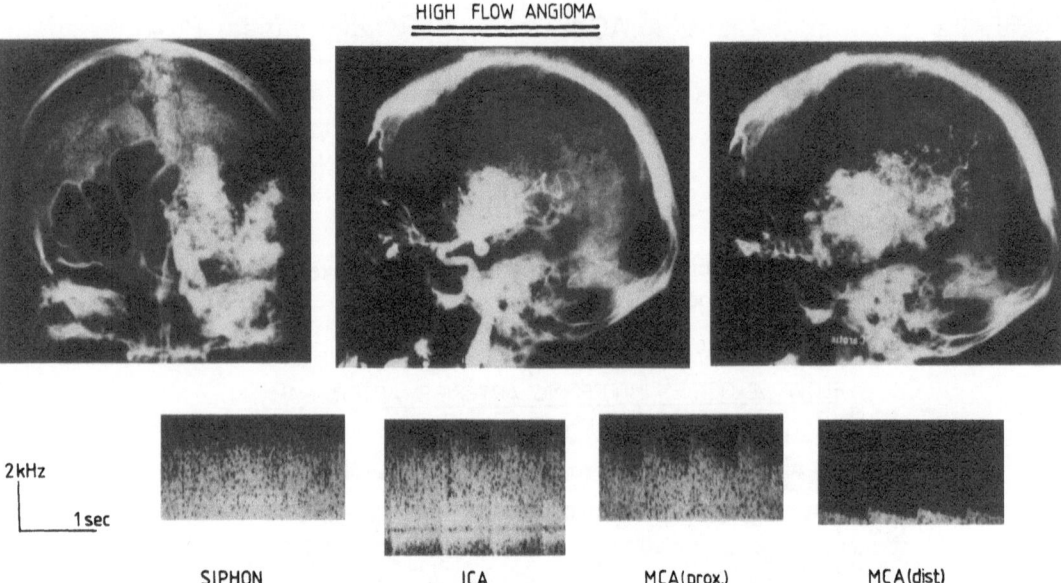

Fig. 92. This angioma can be classified as a high flow angioma. In angiography the
brain arteries are only slightly filled. The velocities in the feeding arteries are very
high, more than 3.6 kHz in diastole, the distal branch of the MCA shows reduced
flow velocities as sign of the steal effect of the angioma

The partial exclusion of the AVM on the 25th day resulted in continuous
reduction of the velocities. After total exclusion, the velocites immediately
dropped to below normal and then gradually reached the normal value.

In the AVM shown in Fig. 92, there are very high velocities accompanied
by musical murmurs, both in the siphon segment and in the supraclinoid
segment of the carotid artery. The velocity of the blood flow from the MCA,
which was identified by Doppler sonography, has risen to 2 ½ times the
normal value, while a peripheral branch of the MCA shows velocities that
have dropped to below normal. This is an indication of reduced perfusion of
the ipsilateral hemisphere caused by the steal effect of the AVM.

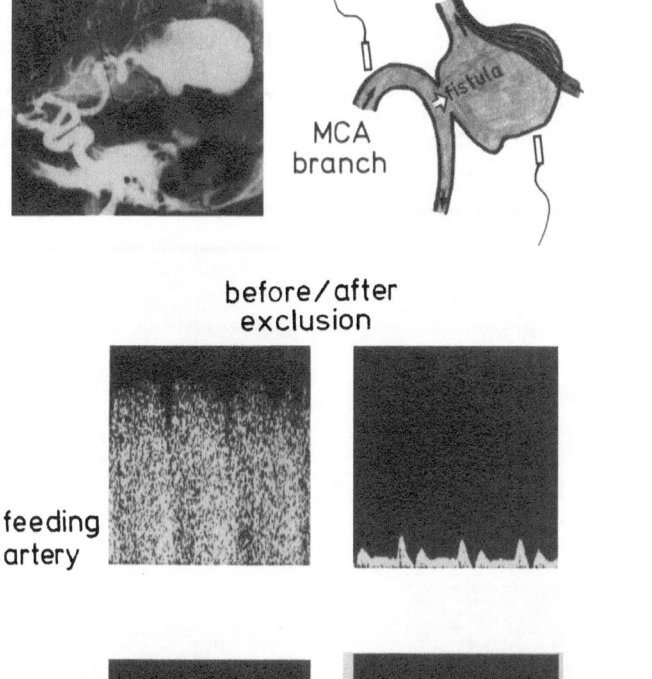

before/after
exclusion

feeding
artery

draining
vein

Fig. 93

ARTERIO-VENOUS FISTULA AND TRANSCRANIAL DOPPLER

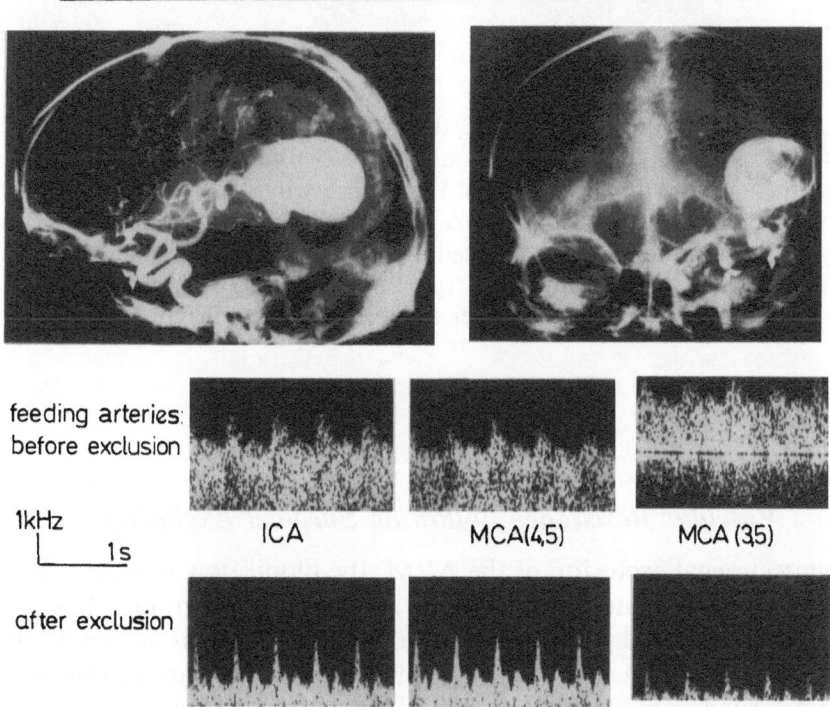

feeding arteries:
before exclusion

1kHz

1s

ICA   MCA(4,5)   MCA (3,5)

after exclusion

Figs. 93 and 94. Intraoperative (Fig. 93) and transcranial (Fig. 94) Doppler investigations of an arteriovenous fistula fed by a branch of the middle cerebral artery with high flow velocities. The high diastolic flow is a sign of reduced peripheral resistance. After exclusion of the angioma, signs of increased resistance in the artery that had originally fed the angioma could be observed

AVM EMBOLIZATION BY SUPERSELECTIVE ARTERIOGRAPHY

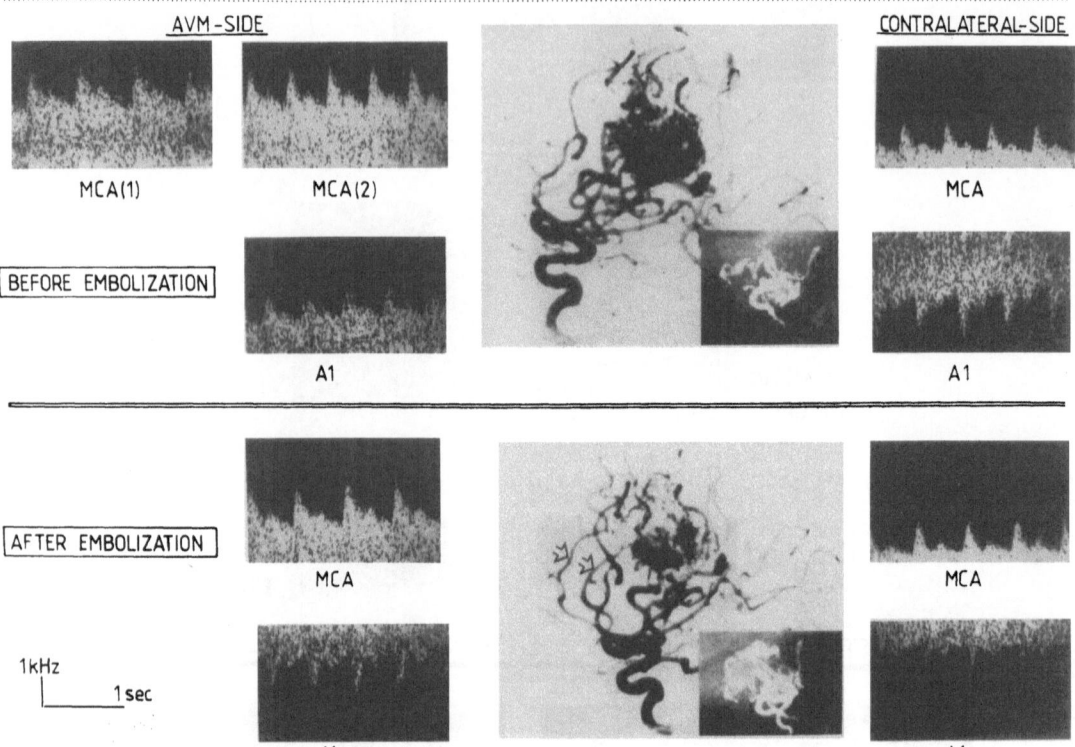

Fig. 95. Prior to the third embolization, the diastolic velocity in the MCA (1) was still increased to more than 2 kHz. A small catheter placed in this artery did not show any hemodynamic effect (MCA 2). There was retrograde flow in the A1 on the angioma side due to the steal effect to the angioma. After embolization, flow velocity in the feeding MCA was reduced, the flow in the A1 became orthograde, and in angiography the pericallosal artery became visible. This is an example of a hemodynamic change after superselective embolization

Vascular Resistance Following Surgical Exclusion

Following surgical exclusion of the AVM, the blood flow velocities in the feeding arteries are immediately reduced. In Doppler sonography they show clear signs of increased peripheral resistance. In the patient in Figs. 93 and 94, a change in the frequency spectra from the internal to external type could be demonstrated by intraoperative Doppler investigation and postoperative transcranial Doppler.

Superselective Embolization and TCD Recordings

With the new thin embolization catheters (outer diameter 0.8 mm, inner diameter 0.4 mm), it is possible to selectively reach feeding arteries in the AVM (Merland). In the case illustrated in Fig. 95, placing the embolization catheter in an AVM vessel does not cause any spastic reaction and thus no measurable change in blood flow velocity.

In this Sylvian angioma, which had already been preembolized, there was a threefold increase in the flow velocities in the MCA. Because of the steal effect of the AVM, the anterior cerebral artery cannot be demonstrated by angiography. The direction of flow in the A1 segment on the side of the AVM is retrograde. After embolization, a marked reduction of velocity occurs in the MCA and there is again orthograde flow in the A1. The pericallosal artery can now be visualized in angiography.

Fig. 96 shows the angiographic and Doppler sonographic findings following two superselective embolization preocedures. There is a continuous reduction of velocities in the precommunicating segment of the posterior cerebral artery, while in the postcommunicating segment of the posterior cerebral artery a velocity decrease occurs after the second embolization.

The embolization of the temporal AVM in Fig. 97 causes no reduction of the velocity in the feeding MCA. The MCA on the opposite side produces a normal frequency spectrum. Neither does the AVM in Fig. 98 show any velocity reduction in the MCA after embolization. The CO_2 reactivity is still considerably limited, particularly in the presence of hypercapnia, as a sign of the embolization effect, which is not yet hemodynamically measurable.

Discussion

Intravascular pressure recordings and measurements of blood flow velocity and volume flow in patients with arteriovenous malformations performed during surgery have confirmed the following hemodynamic principles: [150, 153, 155] the more blood an AMV needs because of the reduced vascular resistance in the shunt system, the wider the lumen of the feeding arteries becomes and the faster the blood flows in these arteries. Intravasal pressure measurements [153] have shown that the intravasal pressure reduction of the feeding arteries, in contrast to the systemic arterial blood pressure, is highest in the vessels that are dilated the most. It has also been established intraoperatively that autoregulation is lacking in the feeding arteries [153]. The high pressure gradient from "normal" blood supply of cerebral tissue to the angioma can cause a cerebral steal effect [56], which leads to hyperfusion of the surrounding brain tissue. A reactive dilatation of the brain vessels lowers the resistance in order to achieve better perfusion.

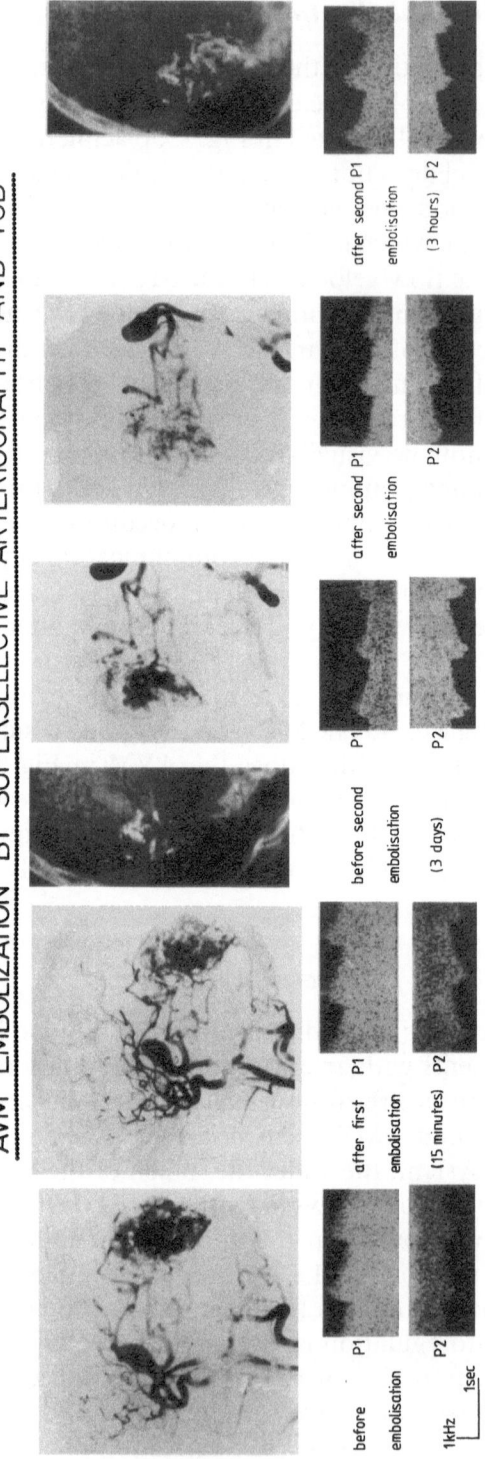

AVM EMBOLIZATION BY SUPERSELECTIVE ARTERIOGRAPHY AND TCD

Fig. 96. This large occipital angioma was superselectively embolized twice: the velocity in the feeding P1 after the second embolization was reduced and the P2 segment showed lowered velocity after the second embolization. Three hours after the second embolization a moderate increase in velocity in the P1 could be observed. This may be due to new AVM anastomoses

AVM EMBOLIZATION BY SUPERSELECTIVE ARTERIOGRAPHY

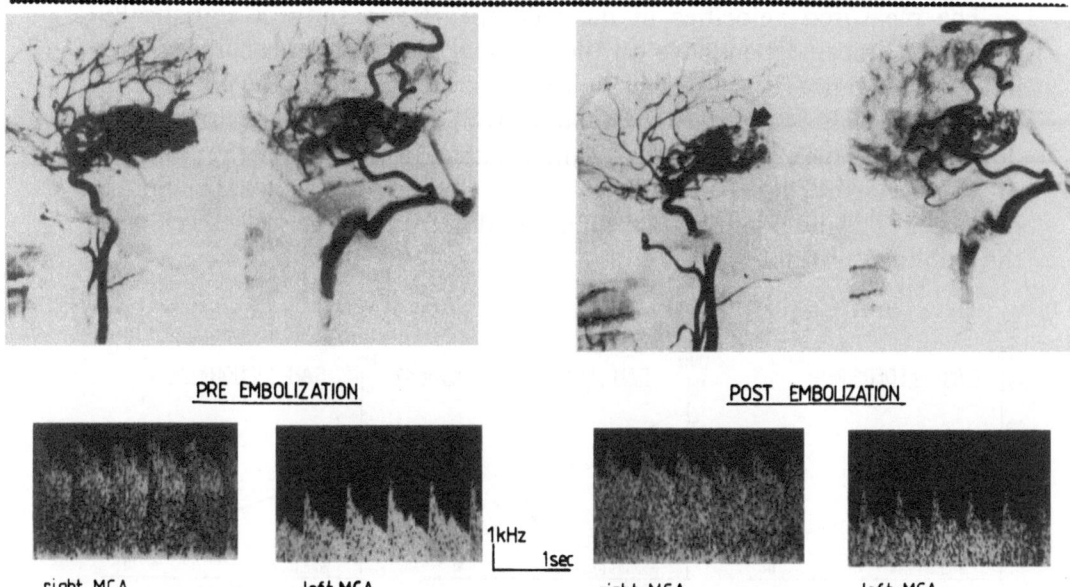

PRE EMBOLIZATION

POST EMBOLIZATION

1kHz

1sec

right MCA   left MCA   right MCA   left MCA

Fig. 97. Superselective embolization of a small part of this temporal angioma did not cause any change in flow velocity in the feeding arteries

AVM EMBOLIZATION BY SUPERSELECTIVE ARTERIOGRAPHY

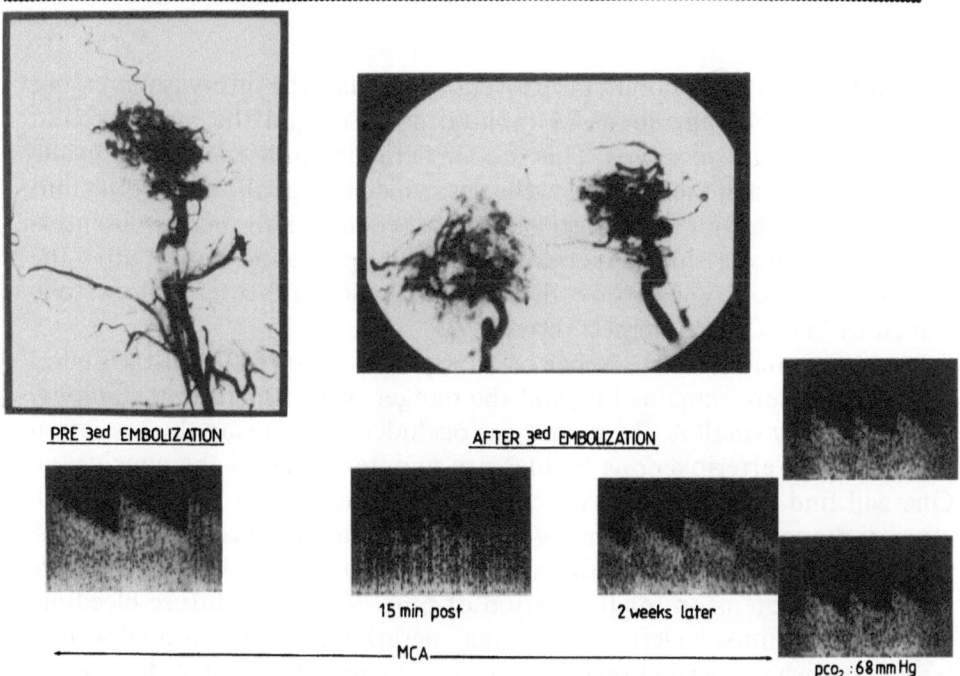

PRE 3ed EMBOLIZATION

AFTER 3ed EMBOLIZATION

15 min post   2 weeks later

MCA

pco_2 : 68 mm Hg

Fig. 98. After the third embolization there were only few velocity changes in the MCA. The CO_2 reactivity was still limited

The measured velocities in the feeding arteries show a statistically significant linear dependence on the vascular resistance measured as the index of resistance (Fig. 99). The highest diastolic velocity in the presence of large AVMs was 4 kHz (in two patients). However, 70% of the patients had diastolic velocities between only 2.2 and 3.4 kHz. In contrast, in the presence of vessel narrowings (spasm, stenosis), velocities up to 6 kHz can be measured. The index of resistance measured in front of the spastic vessel at the siphon is normal.

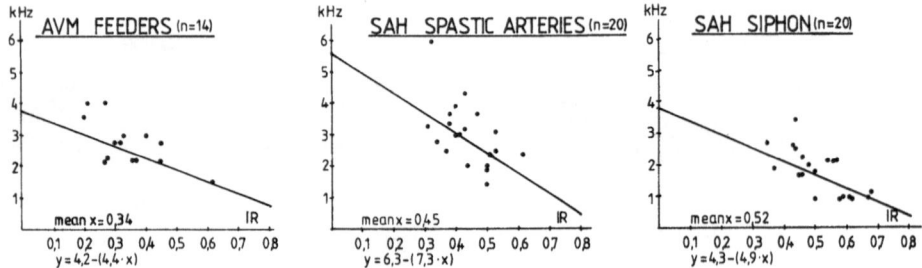

Fig. 99. Blood flow velocities in the feeding arteries in AVMs increase with the reduction of the index of resistance. While the index of resistance measured in the carotid siphon in 20 patients with spastic MCAs or ICAs is normal, the index of resistance in the spastic arteries is slightly reduced

After surgical resection of arteriovenous fistulas, the intravasal pressure in the vessels feeding the AVM rapidly increases and the local cerebral perfusion pressure decreases. This sudden hemodynamic change causes the pulse wave to reach the dilated capillaries, which brings about bleeding into the operative site and the danger of cerebral edema. This increase in intra-arterial pressure is shown in transcranial Doppler sonography after the exclusion of the AVM by low diastolic velocities and brief high systolic velocities (index of resistance above 0.7).

Assuming that in the presence of arteriovenous shunts the intracerebral vascular pressure remains low and the danger of hemorrhage is minimal, small and very small AVM vessels are occluded first during the operation and the large arteriovenous fistulas are maintained until the conclusion. One will find that bleedings which at 120 mm Hg cannot be arrested will stop spontaneously at 100 mm Hg systemic arterial pressure. In these cases, it is necessary to maintain the anesthesia for 12 to 24 hours to ensure artificical hypotension for this period of time. If there is diffuse bleeding, certain shunts must be left open and the operation must be repeated several weeks later when the cerebral vessels have become narrower in order to close the remaining shunts.

Preoperative embolization has gained increasing importance in the last few years. AVMs could formerly only be partially removed by embolization, but today some of them can be totally removed under the superselective application of embolism. The procedure is complicated and requires a great amount of experience on the part of the neuroradiologist (Merland).

These few examples of cases before and after superselective embolization show that the flow velocity in the vessels feeding the AVM decrease slowly and the conversion of shunt flow to perfusion flow takes place slowly. The risk of bleeding and cerebral edema is thus reduced.

From this it can be concluded that in the majority of cases, preoperative embolization with surgical exclusion of the residual angioma should be the method of choice. This is in accordance with the hemodynamic effects of staged surgery.

It is too soon to be able to make a classification of AVMs according to Doppler sonographic criteria. Further experience with Doppler sonography (velocity measurement, measurement of the CO_2 reactivity) will show whether such AVMs that cause a "circulatory breakthrough" (Nornes) when suddenly excluded totally can be detected by this method. The transcranial Doppler sonographic investigation alone is not an adequate method of judging the "activity" of an AVM. It is, however, a helpful supplementary method of obtaining information on the steal phenomenon in the circle of Willis. Angiography will remain indispensable in the diagnosis and control of the therapy of arteriovenous malformations.

Monitoring of Frequency Spectra in the MCA During Angiography

To determine the effect of contrast medium injected during angiographic examinations on the blood flow velocity in the middle cerebral artery, velocities in the MCA were recorded transcranially while contrast agent was being applied. Shortly after 10 ml contrast medium was injected into the cervical carotid artery, a loud noise could be heard in the Doppler sonographic recording, which lasted for 10 seconds. After the autotransfusion of 10 ml blood, the same phenomenon occurred, however, for only 6 seconds (Fig. 100).

These Doppler shift signals could easily be interpreted as a turbulent flow alteration in the MCA caused by the contrast agent or blood injection.

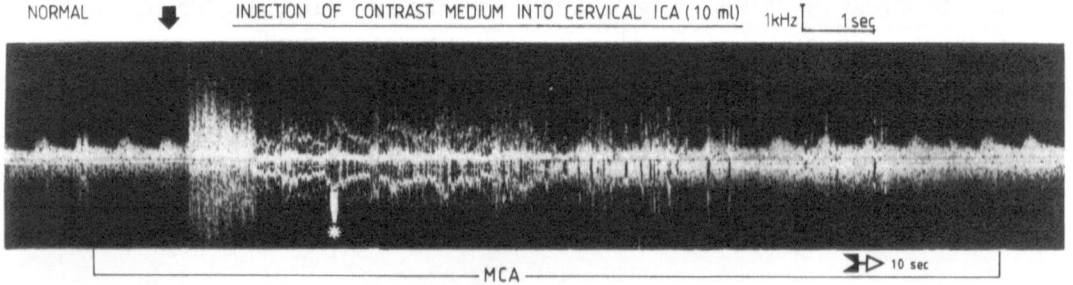

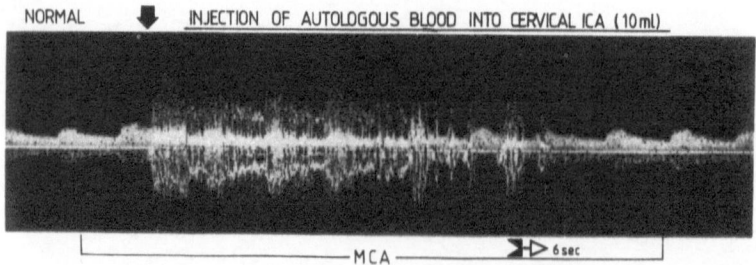

Fig. 100. During the injection of contrast medium or blood into the cervical ICA, noises are registered with high intensity while transcranial Doppler is recording the MCA

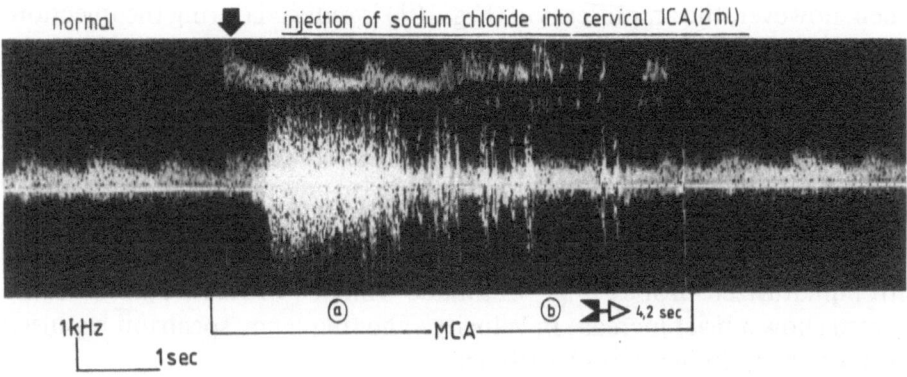

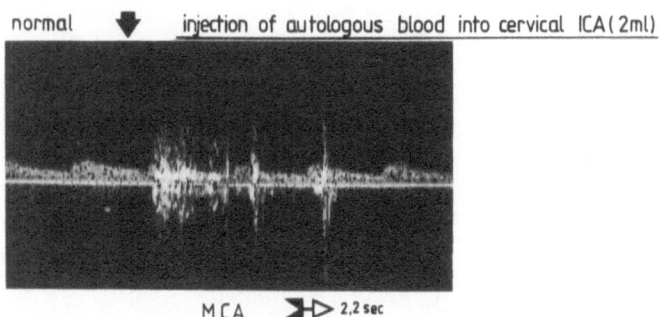

Fig. 101. The same phenomenon could be observed under the injection of 2 ml of sodium chloride or blood. But when the gain of the Doppler machine was reduced during the injection, normal frequency spectra could be recorded in the MCA *a*. In *b* the gain is turned down so low that only few frequencies can be recorded

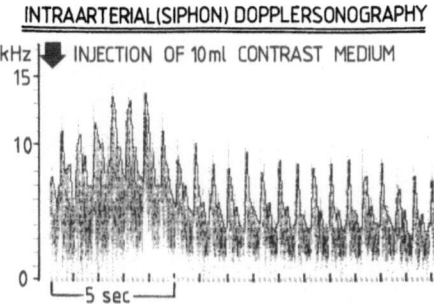

Fig. 102. Recording of flow velocities by intra-arterial Doppler sonography (20 MHz microvascular Doppler). When 10 ml contrast medium were injected there was an increase in velocity, but no signs of turbulence

When, however, the amplification (Fig. 101) is reduced during the injection, a normal pulsed frequency spectrum is obtained with no signs of turbulence.

The interface of the blood and contrast medium increases the back-scattering characteristics of the fluid under ultrasonic examination.

The bands of increased intensity of the frequencies (Fig. 100) are physically caused by harmonic multiples. This effect occurs at amplifier saturation points.

Intravasal Doppler sonographic recordings (20 MHz pulsed Doppler with miniaturized probes, Fig. 102) made while contrast medium is being injected show a brief increase in velocity. The frequency spectrum is pulsed and there is no indication of turbulence.

The injection of contrast medium into cervical brain-supplying arteries has no effect on the laminar pulsed blood flow.

Vascular Hemodynamic Response to Meningitis

Introduction

Vascular stenoses in the large basal cerebral vessels in the presence of tuberculous meningitis were first recognized in angiography by Greitz in 1964 [72]. The angiographic picture of the changes in the vessel lumen of both large and small cerebral vessels was described not only in the case of tuberculous meningitis, but also in purulent meningitis [43, 44, 58, 90, 113, 114, 126]. Pathomorphological findings of these vascular stenoses have been studied by several investigators [38, 44, 72, 178, 211].

In two patients with purulent meningitis, transcranial Doppler sonographic investigations were carried out over a considerable period of time. In the following, the extent to which these angiographic and morphological vascular changes correlate with those described in the literature is discussed.

Case Reports

Case 1: A 26-year-old man suffered an extensive bifrontal basal skull fracture in a traffic accident and developed rhinorrhea and rapidly progressing pneumatocephalus. On September 6, 1985, the direct intracranial repair of the dural fistula was performed. The patient became increasingly drowsy the next few days until coma finally occurred. The CSF showed 130, 000/3 neutrophilic leukocytes, culture revealed pastuerella multocida. After antibiotic therapy and external ventricular drainage, the CSF was free of bacteria by the 20th of September. On September 24 there were renewed clinical signs of meningitis: in the CSF 300/3 white blood cells per mm^3, culture revealed staphylococci. After a massive rhinorrhea occurred again on September 25, the direct intracranial repair of the dural fistula was carrried out. The supraclinoid segment of the right internal carotid artery was narrowed to approximately ⅓ of the normal size. Intraoperative Doppler sonography revealed a marked increase in blood flow velocity. After topical application of nimodipine a moderate arterial dilatation was observed and the flow velocity decreased (Fig. 103). On October 7, a ventriculo-arterial shunt was performed due to hydrocephalus secondary to meningitis.

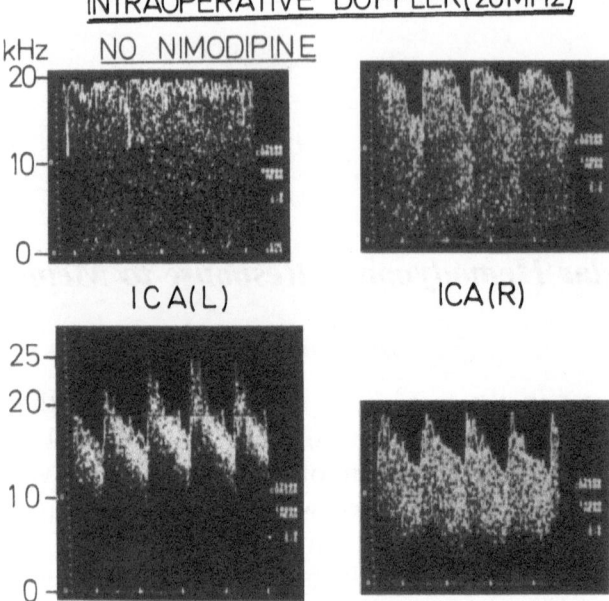

Fig. 103. On the 20th day after the onset of meningitis, the flow velocities in the distal segment of the internal carotid artery on both sides could be recorded by intraoperative Doppler sonography. On the left side the velocities were higher than half the PRF of the machine, which meant that the systolic high velocities could not be recorded. After nimodipine was topically applied, the velocities decreased and the outer diameter of the arteries became slightly dilated

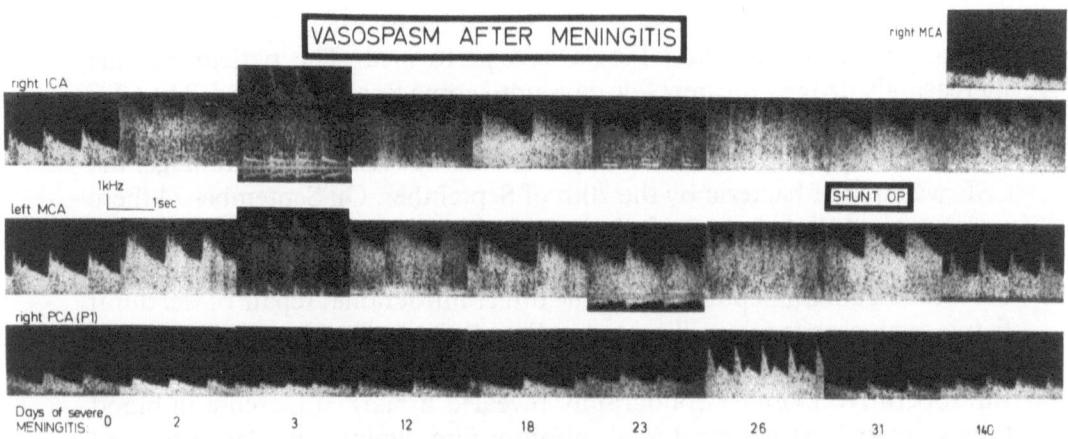

Fig. 104. Severe frequency increase in the right ICA and left MCA in a patient with a severe purulent meningitis. The clinical symptoms of meningitis became worse from day 23 on, at which time TCD again began to record increased flow velocities

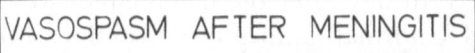

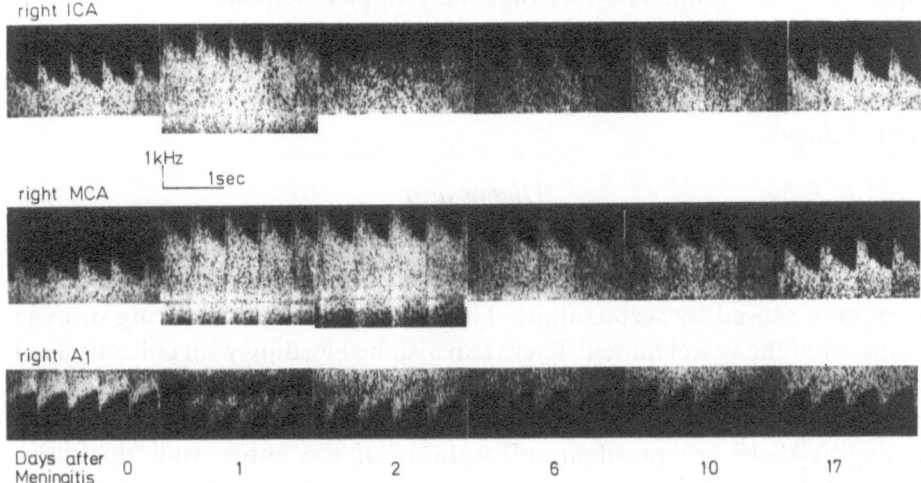

Fig. 105. Rapid increase in flow velocities in the first 2 days after purulent meningitis. Flow pattern returns to normal within 3 weeks

Transcranial Doppler recordings showed an increase in flow velocity both in the right ICA and in the proximal segment of the left MCA within the first three days after the clinical signs of menigitis had appeared (Fig. 104). The velocities in the posterior cerebral artery showed normal velocity. While the blood flow velocities in the left MCA returned to normal 70 days after the onset of meningitis, in the ICA there was an increase up to the 140th day. At the time of the second meningitis attack between the 18th and 23rd day, Doppler sonography again showed increased velocities. The last investigation on the 140th day showed that distal to the spastic carotid artery the velocity in the MCA was reduced to half the normal value. This denotes a hemodynamically effective narrowing in the carotid artery.

Case 2: The 31-year-old patient was operated on in July 1984 for a giant bifrontal parasagittal meningeoma. One year later after a serious attack of influenza with paranasal sinus infection, cerebral seizures occurred. CT showed a fronto-basal brain abscess on the right, which was treated by stereotactic puncture. During this procedure sepsis occurred, making it necessary to remove the ventriculo-arterial shunt. Several hours after shunt removal the patient developed a high fever and in the CSF there were 2,924/3 neutrophilic leukocytes. CSF culture revealed diploccal pneumonia. In connection with the raised temperature due to an onset of meningitis, there were marked frequency increases in the right ICA, MCA, and in the right A1, while on the left side Doppler findings were normal (Fig. 105). With the decrease of pyrexia under treatment with antibiotics up to the 10th day after removal of the shunt, there was a reduction of the Doppler frequencies. On the 17th day after the meningitis had set in the Doppler frequencies returned to normal. Clinically, and in the culture, the meningitis appeared to be cured. The fact that the Doppler frequencies increased to three times the norm within 2 days and then rapidly returned to normal within 2 weeks is probably due to vasospasm. The relatively mild meningitis had led to no permanent hemodynamically effective morphological vascular changes.

Discussion

The histopathological changes of the cerebral arteries following meningitis include [38] a separation of the endothelium from the inner elastic membrane caused by serous fluid. This can result in a narrowing or even occlusion of the vessel lumen. There can also be bleeding with collections of fibrin. Leukocytes cause a purulent endarteritis with swelling of the endothelial cells. An edema of the adventitia forms. In the case of chronic meningitis there are purulent infiltrations of the entire wall thickness, fibroid necroses of the entire vessel wall or only of the intima. After 7–8 weeks, mainly profilerative changes in the vessel wall occur, fibrinoid necroses of the intima or of the entire vessel wall. In the case of both specific and nonspecific meningitis there are marked intima hyperplasia that are rich in cells. This can lead to severe stenoses or even complete occlusion of the vessels. Leeds [113] described both vessel narrowing and vessel enlargement. It is still a matter of frequent discussion as to whether the vessel narrowing established in angiography is caused by the morphological thickening of the arterial wall or by vasospasm.

In Case 1 it was possible to confirm intraoperatively that the outer diameter of the vessel was considerably reduced. Topical application of the calcium antagonist produced a decrease of blood velocity as a result of vessel enlargement. The increase in velocity in the carotid artery lasting 140 days (Fig. 104) cannot be explained by vasoconstriction (vasospasm). Morphological changes in the artery must have led to lumen narrowing.

Since the blood flow velocities in the MCA were considerably reduced, there must have been a hemodynamically critical stenosis in the carotid artery and not a peripheral vasodilatation as a sign of disturbed autoregulation. Improved cerebral perfusion by induced hypertension treatment or by the administration of calcium antagonists in the acute phase of meningitis could result in a reduction of the neurological deficits caused by ischemia. The percentage of peripheral cerebral infarcts diagnosed by computed tomography in the case of tuberculous meningitis is given at 20.5% [36]. As hydrocephalus can occur in 76% after meningitis, the danger of reduced cerebral perfusion is high. Early shunt operation and induced hypertension can improve cerebral perfusion pressure and reduce the incidence and severity of remaining ischemic neurological deficits.

Brain Death and TCD Recordings

Brain death is clinically defined as the complete and irreversible cessation of the total brain function, even though the circulation in the rest of the body continues. The patient is no longer able to breathe spontaneously and must be mechanically ventilated. The death of the brain means the death of the person [207].

To confirm brain death, electroencephalogram or cerebral angiography or both are performed to document the cessation of brain function or brain circulation. Cerebral circulatory cessation occurs when the cerebral perfusion pressure is zero, which means that the arterial blood pressure is the same as the intracranial pressure.

The most reliable method of showing cerebral blood flow arrest is the four-vessel angiography (Fig. 106) [29, 37, 208]. Other less invasive methods are isotope angiography [70] and pulsation echoencephalography [145, 200]. These methods, however, provide less reliable information.

Doppler sonography was able to establish characteristic changes in the flow waveforms of the extracranial brain-supplying arteries in the case of brain death. Studies on the end branches of the opthalmic artery (supratrochlear and supraorbital arteries), however, are not reliable diagnostic measures [143].

In the internal carotid artery and the vertebral artery, there is a marked reduction of the systolic orthograde flow and an early diastolic retrograde phase [33, 34, 118, 213]. The reverberating flow pattern with counterbalancing forward and backward components of the blood column indicates flow arrest. The forward/backward phenomenon found in the internal carotid and vertebral arteries is a result of compliance of the cerebral arteries (Fig. 107).

Transcranial Doppler findings were obtained in 15 patients who fulfilled the clinical criteria for brain death, were mechanically ventilated, and who had a systolic blood pressure between 80 and 120 mm Hg. In all cases reliable Doppler signals could be registered at a measuring depth of 4–5 cm (middle cerebral artery, end segment of the internal carotid artery). All of the patients died within 24 hours or upon discontinuation of the mechanical ventilation. In six cases, the arrest of cerebral blood flow could be verified by angiography.

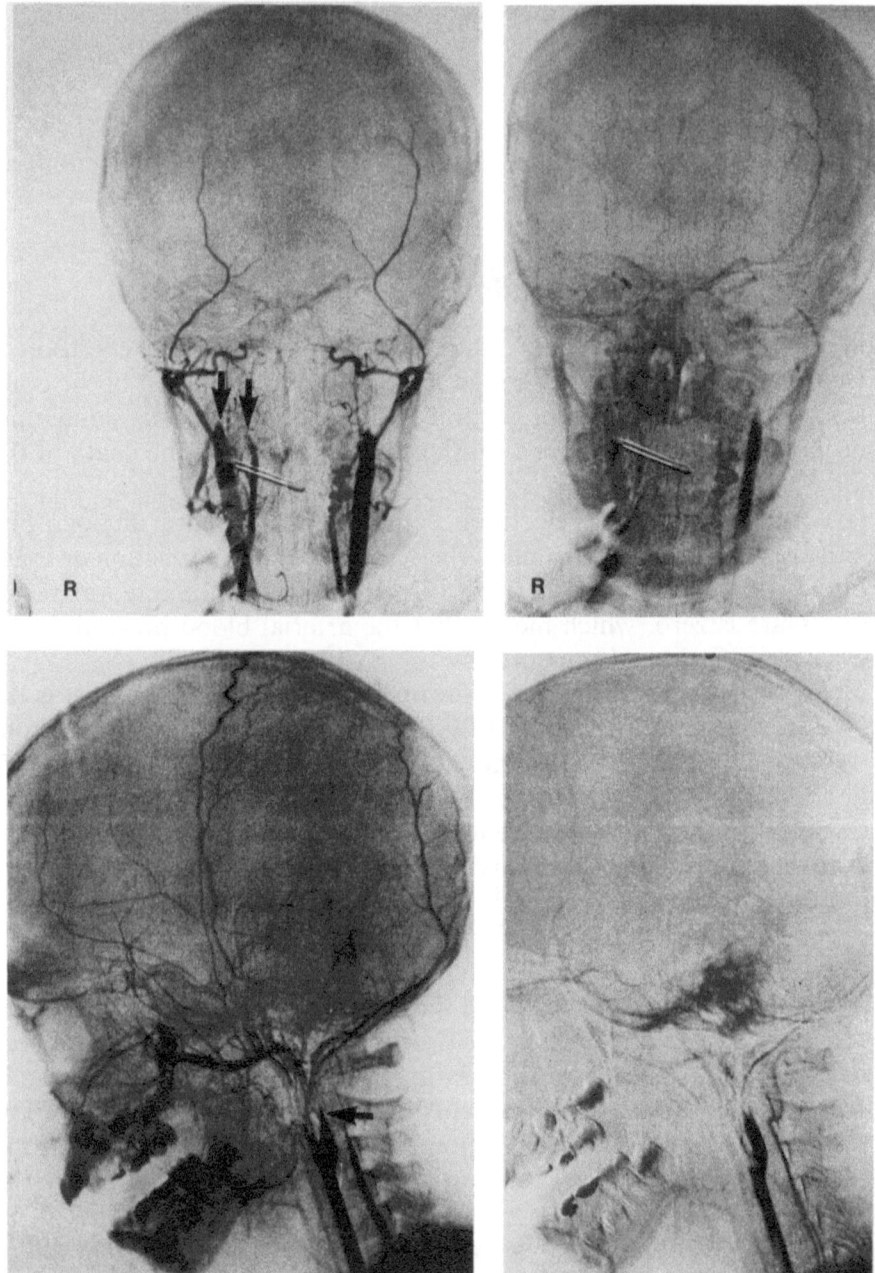

Fig. 106. Angiographic findings in a patient with a severe head injury. No contrast medium in both internal carotid arteries and both vertebral arteries indicating no cerebral perfusion

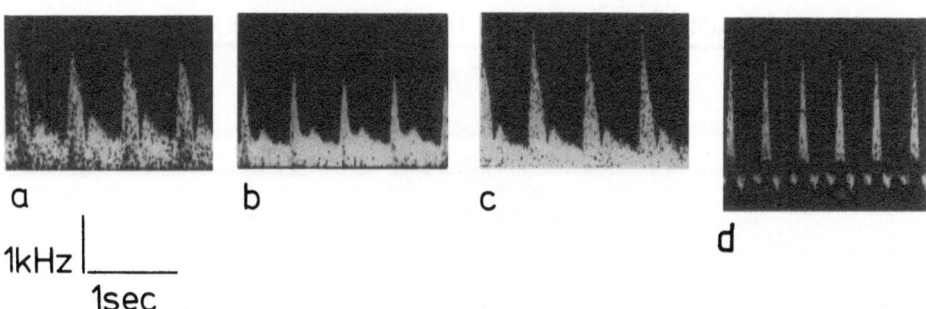

a   b   c

d

1kHz

1sec

Fig. 107. Signs of increased peripheral vescular resistance in transcranial Doppler sonography. *a* Velocity in the MCA of a 74-year-old patient with arteriosclerosis. *b* MCA velocity in a 40-year-old patient without cerebral vascular disease during hyperventilation. *c* Frequency spectra of a 60-year-old patient with increased intracranial pressure up to 170 mm H_2O. He had a hydrocephalus secondary to an aneurysmal subarachnoid hemorrhage. *d* 30-year-old patient who suffered a severe head injury. Only forward and reversed flow could be detected in the MCA as a sign of zero net flow indicating brain death

FLOW VELOCITY PATTERN IN MCA

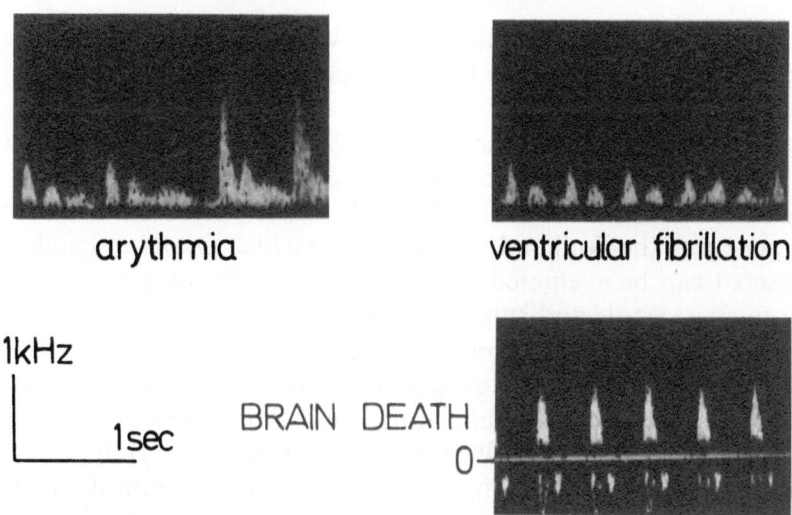

arythmia   ventricular fibrillation

1kHz

1sec   BRAIN DEATH

0

Fig. 108. 36-year-old man suffering spontaneous intracerebral hemorrhage with hematocephalus. At the stage of a midbrain syndrome there were very low time averaged peak frequencies in the MCA during arrhythmia and ventricular fibrillation. There was early diastolic and late diastolic zero flow. Eight hours later the patient showed all clinical signs of brain death and in the Doppler recordings there was reverberating flow pattern in the MCA

BRAIN DEATH AND TRANSCRANIAL DOPPLER

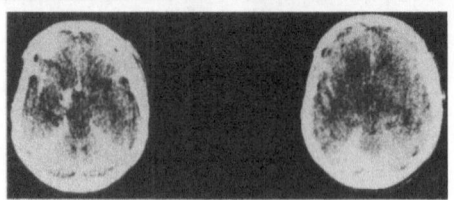

right MCA   inspiration exspiration   left MCA

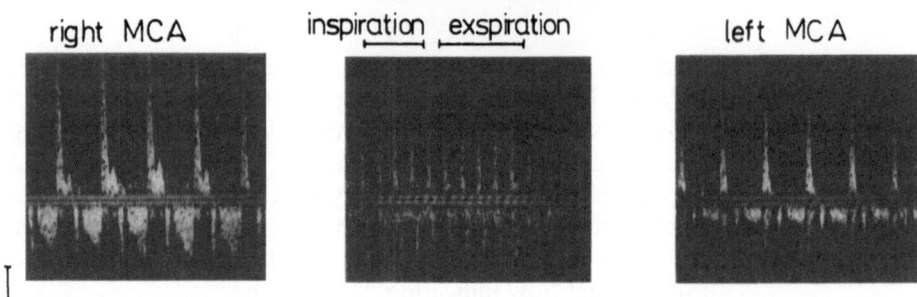

Fig. 109. In this patient the subarachnoid aneurysmal hemorrhage resulted in a severe generalized edema followed by the clinical signs of brain death. The Doppler findings show typical reverberating flow pattern with zero net flow. The change in the frequency shifts induced by the mechanical ventilation is shown

The transcranial Doppler findings showed the same marked forward/backward flow phenomena as those in the extracranial internal carotid artery (Figs. 108 and 109).

Using transcranial Doppler sonography, the phenomenon of early diastolic backward flow in the cervical vessels upon flow arrest can now be established directly on intracranial vessels. Since in 6% the sound beam cannot penetrate the skull, only those cases in which Doppler signals could be registered can be evaluated. Brief orthograde movement of the blood column during systole and subsequent early diastolic retrograde flow are caused by compliance of the cerebral arteries.

Intracranial reverberating flow patterns in the large basal sections of the circle of Willis are a reliable indication of circulatory cerebral blood flow arrest. Further experience will show whether this relatively fast, non-invasive method is able to distinguish between primary brain stem damage and secondary damage caused by supratentorial pressure. Early diagnosis of brain death is important for transplant surgery.

References

1. Aaslid R, Markwalder Th-M, Nornes H (1982) Noninvasive transcranial Doppler ultrasound recording of flow velocity in basal cerebral arteries. J Neurosurg 57: 769–774
2. Aaslid R, Huber P, Nornes H (1984) Evaluation of cerebrovascular spasm with transcranial Doppler ultrasound. J Neurosurg 60: 37–41
3. Aaslid R, Nornes H (1984) Musical murmurs in human cerebral arteries after subarachnoid hemorrhage. J Neurosurg 60: 32–36
4. Allen GS, et al. (1983) Cerebral arterial spasm—a controlled trial of nimodipine in patients with subarachnoid hemorrhage. New Engl J Med 38: 619–624
5. Allock JM, Drake CG (1965) Ruptured intracranial aneurysms—the role of arterial spasm. J Neurosurg 22: 21–29
6. Alvord EC, Thorn RB (1977) Natural history of subarachnoid hemorrhage: early prognosis. Clin Neurosurg 24: 167–175
7. Aoyagi N, Hayakawa I (1984) Analysis of 223 ruptured intracranial aneurysms with special reference to rupture. Surg Neurol 24: 445–452
8. Araujo LC, Zapulla RA, Yang WC, Hollin SA (1978) Angiographic changes to induced hypertension in cerebral vasospasm. J Neurosurg 49: 312–315
9. Arnolds BJ, von Reutern GM (1986) Transcranial Doppler Sonography. Examination-technique and normal reference values. Ultrasound Med Biol 12/2: 115–123
10. Arts MGJ, Roevros JMJG (1972) On the instantaneous measurement of bloodflow by ultrasonic means. Med Biol Engng 10: 23–34
11. Auer LM, Ito Z, Suzuki A, Otha H (1982) Prevention of symptomatic vasospasm by topically applied nimodipine. Acta Neurochir 63: 297–302
12. Auer LM (1984) Acute operation and preventive nimodipine improve outcome in patients with ruptured cerebral aneurysms. Neurosurgery 15: 57–66
13. Auer LM, Suzuki A, Yasui N, Ito Z (1984) Intraoperative topical nimodipine after aneurysm clipping. Neurochirurgia 27: 36–38
14. Austin G, Laffin D, Hayword W (1974) Physiologic factors in the selection of patients for superficial temporal artery-to-middle cerebral artery anastomosis. Surgery 75: 861–868
15. Austin G, Gaskell R (1984) Intracranial aneurysm: A computer model. In: Proceedings of cardiovascular system dynamics society, 1984. Philadelphia, University of Pennsylvania

16. Baethmann A (1984) Pathophysiologie der zerebralen Durchblutungs-störungen beim Vasospasmus. In: Voth D, Glees P (Hrsg) Der zerebrale Angiospasmus. de Gruyter, Berlin New York, S 227–241

17. Baker DW (1970) Pulsed Doppler blood-flow sensing. IEEE Trans Son Ultrason SU 17: 170–185

18. Baker DW (1980) Applications of pulsed Doppler techniques. Radiol Clin North Amer 18: 79–103

19. Baker R (1981) Real-time spectrum analyzer. Microcomputing 48–50

20. Barnet HJM, Peerless SJ, Fox AJ, Valberg B, Peacock J (The EC/IC bypass study group) (1985) The international cooperative study of extra-cranial/intracranial arterial anastomosis (EC/IC bypass study): Methodology and entry characteristics. Stroke 16: 397–406

21. Barnet HJM, Sacket DL, Taylor DW, Peerless SJ, Haynes RB, Gates PC, Fox AJ, Mukherjee J, Valberg B, Hachinski V, Lauzier S, Orgogozo JM (1985) Failure of extracranial-intracranial arterial bypass to reduce the risk of ischemic stroke. New Engl J Med 313: 1191–1199

22. Blackshear Jr, WM, Philipps DJ, Chikos PM, Harley JD, Thiele BL, Strandness DE (1980) Carotid artery velocity patterns in normal and stenotic vessels. Stroke 11: 67–71

23. Blaumanis OR, Grady A, Nelson E (1979) Hemodynamic and morphologic aspects of cerebral vasospasm. In: Price TR, Nelson E (eds) Cerebrovascular diseases. Raven Press, New York

24. Boullin DJ, Tagari Ph, du Boulay G, Atiken V, Hughes JTh (1983) The role of hemoglobin in the etiology of cerebral vasospasm. J Neurosurg 59: 231–236

25. Bradley EL, Sacerio J (1972) The velocity of ultrasonic in human blood under varying physiologic parameters. J Surg Res 12: 290–297

26. Brandt L (1981) Aspects on cerebral vasospasm. A clinical and experimental study. From the Departments of Neurosurgery and Clinical Pharmacology, University of Lund, Lund, Sweden

27. Brawley BW (1969) Determination of superior sagittal sinus patency with an ultrasonic Doppler flow detector in parasagittal meningioma. J Neurosurg 30: 315–316

28. Brisman R, Grossman BL, Correll JW (1979) Accuracy of transcutaneous Doppler ultrasonics in evaluating extracranial vascular disease. J Neurosurg 32: 529–533

29. Bücheler E, Käufer C, Düx A (1970) Zerebrale Angiographie zur Bestimmung des Hirntodes. Fortschr Röntgenstr 113: 278–289

30. Büdingen HJ, von Reutern GM, Freund HJ (1976) Die Differenzierung der Halsgefäße mit der direktionellen Doppler-Sonographie. Arch Psychiat Nervenkr 222: 177–190

31. Büdigen HJ, von Reutern GM, Freund HJ (1977) Diagnosis of cerebro-vascular lesions by ultrasonic methods. Intern J Neurol 11: 206–218

32. Büdingen HJ, Gilsbach J, von Reutern GM (1978) Dopplersonographische Therapie- und Verlaufskontrolle einer katheteroccludierten Cavernosusfistel. Arch Psychiat Nervenkr 226: 19–27

33. Büdingen HJ (1979) Untersuchungsverfahren bei Bewußtlosen: Neurophysiologische Untersuchungen. In: Ahnefeld FW, Bergmann H, Burri C, Dick W, Halmágyi U, Horsli G, Rügheimer E (Hrsg) Der bewußtlose Patient. Springer, Berlin Heidelberg New York

34. Büdingen HJ, von Reutern GM (1979) Atraumatische Vorfelddiagnostik des Hirntodes mit der Doppler-Sonographie. Dtsch Med Wschr 104: 1347–1351

35. Büdingen HJ, von Reutern GM, Freund HJ (1982) Doppler-Sonographie der extrakraniellen Hirnarterien. G Thieme Stuttgart New York

36. Bullock MRR, Welchman JM (1982) Diagnostic and prognostic features of tuberculous meningitis on CT scanning. J Neurol Neurosurg Psychiat 45: 1098–1101

37. Busse O, Vogelsang H (1974) Transfemorale zerebrale Panarteriographie zur Bestimmung des Hirntodes. Fortschr Röntgenstr 121: 630–634

38. Cervos-Navarro J, Schneider H (Redigiert von Ule G) (1980) Entzündliche Erkrankungen der Hirngefäße. In: Durchblutungsstörungen und Gefäßerkrankungen des Zentralnervensystems. Springer, Berlin Heidelberg New York, S 342–347

39. Chater N (1979) Surgical results and measurements of intraoperative flow in microsurgical anastomoses. In: Austin GM (ed) Microsurgical anastomoses for cerebral ischemia. Ch C Thomas, Springfield, Ill, pp 295–304

40. Chayatte D, Rusch N, Sundt ThM (1983) Prevention of chronic experimental cerebral vasospasm with ibiprofen and high-dose methylprednisolone. J Neurosurg 59: 925–932

41. Conway LW, McDonald LW (1972) Structural changes of the intradural arteries following subarachnoid hemorrhage. J Neurosurg 37: 715–723

42. Crowell RM, Electromagnetic flow studies of superficial temporal artery to middle cerebral branch artery bypass graft. In: Austin GM (ed) Microsurgical anastomoses for cerebral ischemia. Ch C Thomas, Springfield, Ill, pp 116–124

43. Davis DO, Taveras JM (1966) Radiological aspects of inflammatory conditions affecting the central nervous system. In: Mosberg WH Jr (ed) Clinical neurosurgery, vol 14. Williams and Wilkins, Baltimore, pp 192–210

44. Davis DO, Dilenge D, Schlaepfer W (1970) Arterial dilatation in purulent meningitis. Case report. J Neurosurg 32: 112–115

45. Diener HC, Voigt K, Dichgans J (1981) Diagnosis of intracranial malformations by Doppler sonography. Neurochirurgia 24: 185–191

46. Djindjian R, Cophignon J, Merland JJ, Houdart R (1973) Embolization by superselective arteriography from the femoral route in neuroradiology review of 60 cases. I. Technique, indications, complications. Neuroradiology 6: 20–26

47. Djindjian R, Cophignon J, Rey A, Theron J, Merland JJ, Houdart R (1973) Superselective arteriographic embolization by the femoral route in neuroradiology. Study of 50 cases. III Embolization in craniocerebral pathology. Neuroradiology 6: 143–152

48. Van Dongen MEH, van Steenhoven AA (1982) Some fluid dynamical aspects of arterial flow. In: Reneman RS, Hoeks APG (eds) Doppler ultrasound in the diagnosis of cerebrovascular disease. Research Studies Press, Chichester, pp 29–58

49. Doppler Ch (1843) Über das farbige Licht der Doppelsterne und einiger anderer Gestirne des Himmels. Abh Kgl Böhm Ges d Wissensch (Prag), S 465–482

50. Earnest F, Forbes G, Sandok BA, Piepgras DG, Faust RJ, Ilstrup DM, Arndt LD (1983) Complications of cerebral angiography prospective assessement of risk. AJNR 4: 1191–1197

51. Ecker A, Riemenschneider PA (1951) Arteriographic demonstration of spasm of the intradural arteries with special reference to saccular arterial aneurysms. J Neurosurg 8: 660–667

52. Ecker A, Riemenschneider PA (1953) Arteriographic evidence of spasm in cerebral vascular disorders. Neurology (Minneapolis) 3: 495–502

53. Eden A (1986) The beginnings of Doppler. In: Aaslid R (ed) Transcranial Doppler sonography. Springer, Wien New York

54. Espinosa F, Weir B, Overton Th, Castor W, Grace M, Boisvert D (1984) A randomized placebo-controlled double-blind trial of nimodipine after SAH in monkeys. J Neurosurg 60: 1167–1175

55. Espinosa F, Weir B, Shnitka T, Overton T, Boisvert D (1984) A randomized placebo-controlled double-blind trial of nimodipine after SAH in monkeys. Part II: Pathological findings. J Neurosurg 60: 1176–1185

56. Feindel W, Yasamoto YL, Hodge CP (1971) Red cerebral veins and the cerebral steal syndrome. Evidence from fluorescein angiography and micro-regional blood flow by radioisotopes during excision of an angioma. J Neurosurg 35: 167–179

57. Felix RW, Sigel B, Gibson RJ, Williams J, Popky GL, Edelstein AL, Justin JR (1976) Pulsed Doppler ultrasound detection of flow disturbances in arteriosclerosis. J Clin Ultrasound 4: 275–282

58. Ferris EJ, Rudikoff JC, Shapiro JH (1968) Cerebral angiography of bacterial infection. Radiology 90: 727–734

59. Fischer CM, Kistler JP, Davis JM (1980) Relation of cerebral vasospasm to subarachnoid hemorrhage visualized by computerized tomographic scanning. Neurosurgery 6: 1–8

60. Fischer CM, Roberson GH, Ojemann RG (1977) Cerebral vasospasm with ruptured saccular aneurysm—the clinical manifestations. Neurosurgery 1: 245–248

61. Fleischer AS, Tindall GT (1980) Cerebral vasospasm following aneurysm rupture. A protocol for therapy and prophylaxis. J Neurosurg 52: 149–152

62. Fox JL, Ko JP (1978) Cerebral vasospasm: A clinical observation. Surg Neurol 10: 269–275

63. Freed D, Hartley CJ, Christman KD, et al (1979) High-frequency pulsed Doppler ultrasound: a new tool for microvascular surgery. J Microsurg 1: 148–153

64. Freund HJ (1965) Ultraschallregistrierung der Pulsation einzelner intrakranieller Arterien zur Diagnostik von Gefäßverschlüssen. Arch Psychiat. Zschr Ges Neurol 207: 247–253

65. Friedrich H, Hänsel-Friedrich G, Seeger W (1980) Intraoperative Doppler-Sonographie an Hirngefäßen. Neurochirurgia 23: 89–98

66. Fujishiro K, Yoshimura S (1982) Haemodynamic changes in carotid blood flow with age. Jikeikai Med J 29: 125–138

67. Fukumori T, Tani E, Maeda Y, Sukenaga A (1983) Effects of prostacyclin and indiomethacin on experimental delayed cerebral vasospasm. J Neurosurg 59: 829–834

68. Furuhata H, Kanno R, Kodaira K, Aoyagi T, Fujishiro K, Hyashi J, Matsumoto H, Yoshimura S (1978) An ultrasonic blood flow measuring system to detect the absolute volume flow. Jpn J Med Electron Biol Eng 16, Suppl: 334 (in japanese)

69. Gilsbach JM (1983) Intraoperative Doppler sonography in neurosurgery. Springer, Wien New York

70. Goodman JM, Heck LL, Moore BD (1985) Confirmation of brain death with portable isotope angiography: A review of 204 consecutive cases. Neurosurgery 16: 492–497

71. Graf CJ, Perret GE, Torner JC (1983) Bleeding from cerebral arteriovenous malformations as part of their natural history. J Neurosurg 58: 331–337

72. Greitz T (1964) Angiography in tuberculous meningitis. Acta Radiol 2: 369–378

73. Grubb RL, Ratcheson RA, Raichle ME, Klieforth AB, Gado MH (1979) Regional cerebral blood flow and oxygen utilization in superficial temporal-middle cerbral artery anastomosis patients. An exploratory definition of clinical problems. J Neurosurg 50: 733–741

74. Guggiari M, Dagreou F, Rivierez M, Mottet P, Gallais S, Philippon J, Viars P (1984) Prediction of cerebral vasospasm. Value of fibrinogen degradation products (FDP) in the cerebro-spinal fluid (CSF) for prediction of vasospasm following subarachnoid haemorrhage due to a ruptured aneurysm. Acta Neurochir 73: 25–33

75. Hamer J (1982) The significance of cerebral vasospasm with regard to early delayed aneurysm surgery. Preliminary results of early surgery. Acta Neurochir 63: 209–213

76. Handa H, Niimi H, Moritake K, Okumura A, Matsuda I, Hayashi K (1977) Analysis of sound spectographic pattern for assessment of vascular occlusive disorders by continuous wave ultrasonic Doppler flowmeter. Arch Jpn Chir 46: 214–225

77. Handa H, Moritake K, Nagata J, et al (1980) Intraoperative hemodynamic study by Doppler ultrasonic flowmeter in the extracranial-intracranial arterial bypass. In: Peerless SJ, Mc Cormick CM (eds) Microsurgery for cerebral ischemia. Springer, Berlin Heidelberg New York, pp 99–105

78. Hartley CJ (1979) Extending the velocity limits of pulsed Doppler ultrasound. 32nd ACEMB, Denver

79. Hartley CJ (1981) Resoluton of frequency aliases in ultrasonic pulsed Doppler velocimeters. IEEE Trans Son Ultrason 28: 69–75

80. Hashi K, Meyer JS, Shinmaru S, Welch KMA, Teraura T (1972) Cerebral hemodynamic and metabolic changes after experimental subarachnoid hemorrhage. J Neurol Sci 17: 1–14

81. Hashimoto T (1984) Dynamic measurement of pressure and flow velocities in glass and silastic model berry aneurysms. Neurol Res 6: 22–28

82. Histand MB, Miller ChW (1972) A comparison of velocity profiles measured in unexposed and exposed arteries. ISA BM 72323: 121–124

83. Hopman H, Gratzl O, Schmiedek P, Schneider I (1977) Doppler sonographic control of microvascular bypass function. In: Schmiedek P, Gratzl O, Spetzler RF (eds) Microsurgery for stroke. Springer, Berlin Heidelberg New York, pp 230–232

84. Hourihan M, Gates PC, McAllister VL (1984) Subarachnoid hemorrhage in childhood and adolescence. J Neurosurg 60: 1163–1166

85. Huber P, Handa J (1967) Effect of contrast material, hypercapnia, hyperventilation, hypertonic glucose and papaverine on the diameter of the cerebal arteries. Invest Radiol 2: 17–32

86. Huckman MS, Shenk GJ, Neems RL, Tiper T (1979) Transfemoral cerebral arteriography versus direct percutaneous carotid and brachial arteriography: A comparison of complication rates. Radiology 132: 93–97

87. Hughes JT, Schianchi PM (1978) Cerebral artery spasm. J Neurosurg 48: 515–525

88. Hunt EW, Hess RM (1968) Surgical risk as related to time of intervention in the repair of intracranial aneurysms. J Neurosurg 28: 14–19

89. Hyodo A, Mizukami M, Kawase T, Nagata K, Yunoki K, Yamaguchi K (1984) Postoperative evaluation of extracranial-intracranial arterial bypass by means of ultrasonic quantitative flow measurement and computed mapping of the electroencephalogram. Neurosurgery 15: 381–385

90. James AE Jr, Hodges FJ, Jordan CE, Mathews EH, Heller R Jr (1972) Angiography and cisternography in acute meningitis duo to Hemophilus influence. Radiology 103: 601–606

91. Jane JA, Kassell NF, Torner JC, Winn HR (1985) The natural history of aneurysms and arteriovenous malformations. J Neurosurg 62: 321–323

92. Jorgensen JE, Campau DN, Baker DW (1973) Physical characteristics and mathematical modelling of the pulsed ultrasonic flowmeter. Med Biol Eng 12, 404–429

93. Kaliman J, Lederbauer M, Fuchs J, Deutsch M, Valencak E (1981 Falsch-negative und falsch-positive Ergebnisse der Karotis-Dopplersonographie — Häufigste Fehlinterpretationen. Ultraschall 2: 141–144

94. Kaneko J, Shiraishi J, Omizo H (1970) Analysis of ultrasonic blood rheogram by the sound spectrograph. Jap Circul 34: 1035–1045

95. Kaneko J, Shiraishi J, Omizo H (1965) An analysing method of ultrasonic blood-rheography with sonography. Digest of the 6th international conference on medical electronics and biological engineering, Tokyo, pp 286–287

96. Kapp JP, Neill WR, Neill ChL, Hodges LR, Smith RR (1982) The three phases of vasospasm. Surg Neurol 18: 40–45

97. Kassell NF, Boarini DJ (1980) Patients with ruptured aneurysm: Pre- and postoperative management. In: Wilkins RA (ed) Cerebral arterial spasm. Williams and Wilkins, Baltimore London

98. Kaye AH, Tagari PhC, Teddy PJ, Adams ChBT, Blaso WP, Boullin DJ (1984) CSF smooth-muscle constrictor activity associated with cerebral vasospasm and mortality in SAH patients. J Neurosurg 60: 927–934

99. Kazda S, Toward R (1982) Nimodipine: a new calcium antagonistic drug with a preferential cerebrovascular action. Acta Neurochir 63: 259–265

100. Keller H (1986) Die cerebrovaskuläre Doppler-Ultraschall-Untersuchung (CW-Doppler) Bull Schweiz Akad Med Wiss 36: 129–142

101. Keller HM, Meier WE, Anlicker M (1976) Noninvasive velocity profile determination in the common carotid artery by means of pulsed Doppler ultrasound. Biomedizin Techn 21: 173

102. Kelly PJ, Gorten RJ, Grossman RG, Eisenberg HM (1977) Cerebral perfusion, vascular spasm, and outcome in patients with ruptured intracranial aneurysms. J Neurosurg 47: 44–49

103. Kodama N, Mizoi K, Sakurai Y, Suzuki J (1980) Incidence and onset of vasospasm. In: Wilkins RA (ed) Cerebral arterial spasm. Williams and Wilkins, Baltimore London

104. Koenig W, Dunn HK, Lacy LY (1946) The sound spectrograph. J Acoust Soc Amer 18: 19–49

105. Kosteljanetz M (1984) CSF of dynamics in patients with subarachnoid and/or intraventricular hemorrhage. J Neurosurg 60: 940–946

106. Kosugi Y, Goto T, Ikebe J, Joshita H, Takakura K (1983) Sonic detection of intracranial aneurysm and AVM. Stroke 14: 37–42

107. Kudo T, Suzuki S, Iwabuchi T (1984) Importance of monitoring the circulation blood volume in patients with cerebral vasospasm after subarachnoid hemorrhage. Neurosurgery 5: 514–520

108. Lang J (1981) Klinische Anatomie des Kopfes. Neurokranium, Orbita, kraniozervikaler Übergang. Springer, Berlin Heidelberg New York

109. Von Lanz, W (1979) Praktische Anatomie, Teil B: Gehirn und Augenschädel. Springer, Berlin Heidelberg New York

110. Lassen NA (1964) Autoregulation of cerebral blood flow. Circ Res 15, Suppl: 201–204

111. Lassen NA, Christensen MS (1976) Physiology of cerebral blood flow. Br J Anaesth 48: 715–734

112. Lassen NA, Astrup J (1985) Cerebrovascular physiology. In Fein L (ed) Cerebrovascular surgery, vol I, pp 75–87

113. Leeds NE, Goldberg HI (1971) Angiographic manifestations in cerebral inflammatory disease. Radiology 98: 595–604

114. Lehrer H (1966) The angiographic triad in tuberculous meningitis. A radiographic and clinicopathologic correlation. Radiology 87: 829–835

115. Leitgeb N, Schuy S (1981) Physikalisch-technische Aspekte der Ultraschalldiagnostik. Ultraschall 2: 185–188

116. Lexell L (1955) Echo-encephalography I. Detection of intracranial complications following head injury. Acta Chir Scand 110: 255–259

117. Liljeqvist L, Ekeström S, Nordhus O (1977) Vergleiche der Doppler-Ultraschallbefunde mit Angiographie-Befunden, intra-operative Druckdifferenzen und Blutflußverhältnissen in der Karotischirurgie. Thoraxchirurgie 25: 266–271

118. Lindegaard KF, Grip A, Nornes H (1980) Precerebral haemodynamics in brain tamponade. Part 1: Clinical studies on blood flow velocity. Neurochirurgia 23: 133–142

119. Linder M (1983) Inhibition by dipyridamole of cerebral vasospasm induced in vitro by whole blood. J Neurosurg 58: 352–355

120. Little JR, Yamamoto YL, Feindel W, *et al* (1979) Superficial temporal artery to middle cerebral artery anastomosis; intraoperative evaluation by fluorescein angiography and xenon-133 clearance. J Neurosurg 50: 560–569

121. Ljunggren B, Brandt L (1982) The outcome in 100 consecutive cases of early aneurysm surgery. Acta Neurochir 63: 215–219

122. Ljunggren B, Brandt L, Säveland H, Nilson PE, Cronqvist St, Andersson KE, Vinge E (1984) Outcome in 60 consecutive patients treated with early aneurysm operation and intravenous nimodipine. J Neurosurg 61: 864–873

123. Ljunggren B, Säveland H, Brand L (1984) Aneurysmal subarachnoid hemorrhage—historical background from a Scandinavian horizon. Surg Neurol 22: 605–616

124. Luessenhop AJ, Presper JH (1975) Surgical embolization of cerebral arteriovenous malformations through internal carotid and vertebral arteries. J Neurosurg 42: 443–451

125. Luessenhop AJ (1984) Natural history of cerebral arteriovenous malformations. In: Wilson ChB, Stein BM (eds) Intracranial arteriovenous malformations. William and Wilkins, Baltimore London, pp 12–23

126. Lyons ED, Leeds NE (1967) The angiographic demonstration of arterial vascular disease in purulent meningitis. Report of a case. Radiology 88: 935–938

127. Macpherson PC, Meldrum SJ, Tunstall-Pedoe DS (1980) A real-time spectrum analyser for ultrasonic Doppler signals, using a chirp-z-transform technique. J Med Eng Tech 4: 24–26

128. Mani RL, Eisenberg RL, McDonald EJ, Pollack JA, Mani JR (1978) Complications of catheter arteriography: Analysis of 5000 procedures. I. Criteria and incidence. Am J Roentgenol 131: 861–865

129. Mani RL, Eisenberg AL (1978) Complications of catheter cerebral arteriography: Analysis of 5,000 procedures. II. Relation of complications rates to clinical and arteriographic diagnoses. Am J Roentgenol 131: 867–869

130. Markwalder TM, Grolimund P, Seiler RW, Roth F, Aaslid R (1984) Dependency of blood flow velocity in the middle cerebral artery on the end-tidal carbon dioxide partial pressure—a transcranial ultrasound Doppler study. J Cereb Blood Flow Metab 4: 368–372

131. Maroon JC, Pieroni DW, Campbell RL (1969) Ophtalmosonometry. An ultrasonic method for assessing carotid blood flow. J Neurosurg 30: 238–246

132. Matjasko MJ, Williams JP, Fontanilla M (1975) Intraoperative use of Doppler to detect successful obliteration of carotid-cavernous fistulas. J Neurosurg 43: 634–636

133. McKusik VA, Murray GE, Peeler RG, Webb GN (1955) Musical murmurs. Bull Johns Hopkins Hosp 97: 136–176

134. Meier WE, Keller H (1976) Der Wert intraopartativer Karotis-Doppler-Sonographie im Hinblick auf Prognose bzw. postoperativen Verlauf. Helv Chir Acta 43: 107–110

135. Merland JJ, Riche MC, Chiras J, Bories J (1981) Therapeutic angiography in neuroradiology. Classical Data, recent advances and perspectives. Neuroradiology 21: 111–121

136. Meyer CHA, Lowe D, Meyer M, Richardson PL, Neil-Dwyer G (1983) Progressive change in cerebral blood flow during the first three weeks after subarachnoid hemorrhage. Neurosurgery 12: 58–76

137. Miyazaki M, Kato K (1965) Measurement of cerebral blood flow by ultrasonic Doppler technique. Jap Circul J 29: 375–382

138. Moritake K, Handa H, Yonekawa Y, Takebe Y, Kishimoto S, Makimoto K (1981) Ultrasonic Doppler Assessment of Hemodynamics in gradual carotid ligation. Stroke 12: 177–182

139. Moritake K, Handa H, Yonekawa Y, et al (1980) Ultrasonic Doppler assessment of hemodynamics in superficial temporal artery-middle cerebral artery anastomosis. Surg Neurol 13: 249–257

140. Muchaidze YuA, Syutkina EV (1979) Determination of the linear velocity of the cerebral blood flow in premature infants. Hum Physiol 5: 595–599

141. Müller HR (1971) Direktionelle Dopplersonographie der A. frontalis medialis. ZEEG, EMG 2: 24–32

142. Müller HR (1972) The diagnosis of internal carotid artery occlusion by directional Doppler sonography of the ophthalmic artery. Neurology (Minneap) 22: 816–832

143. Müller HR (1973) Directional Doppler sonography. A new technique to demonstrate flow reversal in the ophthalmic artery. Neuroradiology 5: 91–94

144. Müller HR, Gratzl O (1980) Quantitative Funktionsprüfung des ATS/ACM/Bypasses mittels eines neuartigen Ultraschall-Flowmeters. Ultraschall 1: 217–222

145. Müller HR (1973) Ultraschalldiagnostik und Hirntodsyndrom. In: Kösl W, Scherzer E (Hrsg) Die Bestimmung des Hirntodzeitpunktes. Maudrich, Wien, S 171–176

146. Newhouse VL, le Cong P, Furgason ES, HoCT (1980) On increasing the range of pulsed Doppler systems for blood flow measurement. Ultrasound Med Biol 6: 233–237

147. Nornes H, Magnaes B (1972) Intracranial pressure in patients with ruptured saccular aneurysm. J Neurosurg 36: 537–547

148. Nornes H, Wikeby P (1977) Cerebral arterial blood flow and aneurysm surgery. Part 1: Local arterial flow dynamics. J Neurosurg 47: 810–818

149. Nornes H, Angelsen B, Lindegaard K-F (1977) Precerebral arterial blood flow pattern in intracranial hypertension with cerebral blood flow arrest. Acta Neurochir 38: 187–194

150. Nornes H, Grip A, Wikeby P (1979) Intraoperative evaluation of cerebral hemodynamics using directional Doppler technique. Part 1: Arteriovenous malformations. J Neurosurg 50: 145–151

151. Nornes H, Grip A, Wikeby P (1979) Intraoperative evaluation of cerebral hemodynamics using directional Doppler technique. Part 2: Saccular aneurysm. J Neurosurg 50: 570–577

152. Nornes H, Lundar T, Wikeby P (1979) Cerebral arteriovenous malformations; results of microsurgical management. Acta Neurochir 50: 243–257

153. Nornes H, Grip A (1980) Hemodynamic aspects of cerebral arteriovenous malformations. J Neurosurg 53: 456–464

154. Nornes H, Grip A (1981) Studies of hemodynamic effects of the exclusion of cerebral arterio-venous malformations. Acta Neurochir 56: 134

155. Nornes H (1984) Quantitation of altered hemodynamics. In: Wilson CB, Stein BM (eds) Intracranial arteriovenous malformations. Williams and Wilkins, Baltimore London, pp 32–43

156. Olinger ChP, Wassermann JF (1977) Electronic stethoscope for detection of cerebral aneurysm, vasospasm and arterial disease. Surg Neurol 8: 298–312

157. Pellettieri L, Carlsson C-A, Grevsten S, Norlen G, Uhlemann Ch (1980) Surgical versus conservative treatment of intracranial arteriovenous malformations. A study in surgical decision-making. Acta Neurochir, Suppl 29

158. Perret G, Nishioka H (1966) An analysis of the diagnostic value and complications of carotid and vertebral angiography in 5484 patients. J Neurosurg 25: 98–114

159. Perret G, Nichioka H (1966) Report on the cooperative study of intracranial aneurysm and subarachnoid hemorrhage. Section VI. Arteriovenous malformations. An analysis of 545 cases of cranio-cerebral arteriovenous malformations and fistulae reported to the cooperative study. J Neurosurg 25: 467–490

160. Pourcelot L (1976) Diagnostic ultrasound for cerebral vascular disease. In: Donald J, Levis S (eds) Present and future of diagnostic ultrasound. Kooyker Scientific Publications, Rotterdam, pp 141–147

161. Pritz MB, Giannotta StL, Kindt GW, McGillicuddy JE, Prager RL (1978) Treatment of patients with neurological deficits associated with cerebral vasospasm by intravascular volume expansion. Neurosurgery 3: 364–368

162. Reivich M (1964) Arterial PCO_2 and cerebral hemodynamics. Am J Physiol 206: 25–35

163. Reneman RS, Hoeks APG (eds) (1982) Doppler ultrasound in the diagnostic of cerebrovascular disease. Research Studies Press

164. Von Reutern G-M, Büdingen HJ, Hennerici M, Freund HJ (1976) Diagnose und Differenzierung von Stenosen und Verschlüssen der Arteria carotis mit der Doppler-Sonographie. Arch Psychiat Nervenkr 222: 191–207

165. Von Reutern G-M, Bündigen HJ, Freund H-J (1976) Dopplersonographische Diagnostic von Stenosen und Verschlüssen der Vertebralarterien und des Subclavian-Steal-Syndroms. Arch Psychiat Nervenkr 222: 209–222

166. Von Reutern G-M, Voigt K, Ortega-Suhrkamp E, et al (1977) Dopplersonographische Befunde bei intrakraniellen vaskulären Störungen: Differentialdiagnose zu Obliterationen der extrakraniellen Hirnarterien. Arch Psychiatr Nervenkr 223: 1891–1896

167. Von Reutern G-M, Büdingen HJ, Ortega-Suhrkamp E, Voigt K, Freund H-J (1978) Differenzierungsmöglichkeiten der extrakraniellen Hirngefäße mit der Ultraschall-Doppler-Sonographie. In: Kriessmann A, Bollinger A (Hrsg) Ultraschall-Doppler Diagnostik in der Angiologie. G Thieme, Stuttgart, S 105–113

168. Von Reutern G-M, Pourcelot L (1978) Cardiac cycle-dependent alternating flow in vertebral arteries with subclavian artery stenoses. Stroke 9: 229–236

169. Von Reutern G-M, Büdingen HJ (1981) Möglichkeiten und Grenzen der Dopplersonographie an den extrakraniellen Hirnarterien. Ultraschall 2: 35–42

170. Ringelstein EB (1984) Ultraschalldiagnostik am vertebro-basilären Kreislauf. 1. Diagnose intrakranieller vertebro-basilärer Thrombosen mit Hilfe der konventionellen Doppler-Sonographie. Ultraschall 5: 215–223

171. Roberts VC, Sainz AJ (1981) Reduction of operator fatigue in Doppler ultrasound blood flow investigations. J Biomed Engng 3: 140–142

172. Rutherford RB, Hiatt WR, Kreutzer EW (1977) The use of velocity wave form analysis in the diagnosis of carotid artery occlusive disease. Surgery 82: 695–702

173. Saito J, Sano K (1980) Vasospasm after aneurysm rupture: Incidence, onset and course. In: Wilkins RH (ed) Cerebral arterial spasm. Williams and Wilkins, Baltimore London, pp 294–301

174. Sano K, Saito I (1978) Timing and indication of surgery of ruptured intracranial aneurysms with regard to cerebral vasospasm. Acta Neurochir 41: 49–60

175. Sasaki T, Asano T, Takakura K, Sano K, Kassell NF (1984) Nature of the vasoactive substance in CSF from patients with subarachnoid hemorrhage. J Neurosurg 60: 1186–1191

176. Satomura Sh (1959) Study of flow patterns in peripheral arteries by ultrasonics. J Acoust Soc Japan 15: 151–158

177. Satomura S, Kaneko Z (1960) Ultrasonic blood rheography. Proceedings of III international conference on med electronics. JEE, London, pp 254–258

178. Schleussing H, Der mikroskopische Befund an den intrameningealen Blutgefäßen bei der Leptomeningitis. In: Bieling R, Bochnik H, et al (Hrsg) Nervensystem, Teil 2: Erkrankungen des zentralen Nervensystems II, Bandteil A. Springer, Berlin Göttingen Heidelberg, S 44–47

179. Seeger W (1978) Atlas of topographical anatomy of the brain and surrounding structures. Springer; Wien New York

180. Seeger W (1980) Microsurgery of the brain 1. Springer, Wien New York

181. Seeger W (1980) Microsurgery of the brain 2. Springer, Wien New York

182. Seeger W (1984) Microsurgery of cerebral veins. Springer, Wien New York

183. Seeger W (1985) Differential approaches in microsurgery of the brain. Springer, Wien New York

184. Smith RR, Yoshioka J (1985) Intracranial arterial spasm. In: Wilkins RH, Rengachary SS (eds) Neurosurgery. McGraw-Hill, pp 1355–1362

185. Smith RR, Clower BR, Grotendurst GM, Yabuno N, Cruse JM (1985) Arterial wall changes in early human vasospasm. Neurosurgery 16: 171–176

186. Sokoloff L (1960) The effects of carbon dioxide on the cerebral circulation. Anesthesiology 21: 664–673

187. Solomon RA, Posst KD, McMurtry III JG (1984) Depression of circulating blood volume in patients after subarachnoid hemorrhage: implications for the management of symptomatic vasospasm. Neurosurgery 15: 354–361

188. Spencer MP, Reid JM (1979) Quantitation of carotid stenosis with continous-wave (C-W) Doppler ultrasound. Stroke 10: 326–330

189. Spencer MP (1981) Blood flow arteries. In: Spencer MP, Reid JM (eds) Cerebrovascular evaluation with Doppler ultrasound. Martinus Nijhoff Publishers, The Hague Boston London, pp 97–112

190. Spencer MP, Reid JM (eds) (1981) Cerebrovascular evaluation with Doppler ultrasound. Martinus Nijhoff, Publishers, The Hague Boston London

191. Spencer MP (1981) Vascular murmurs. In: Spencer MP, Reid JM (eds) Cerebrovascular evaluation with Doppler ultrasound. Martinus Nijhoff, Publishers, The Hague Boston London, pp 89–95

192. Spencer MP, Whisler GD (1985) Transcranial pulsed Doppler for evaluation of cerebral arterial occlusive disease. Stroke 16: 148

193. Spetzler RF, Wilson CB, Weinstein P, Mehdorn M, Townsend J, Telles D (1978) Normal perfusion pressure breakthrough theory. Clin Neurosurg 25: 651–672

194. Steiger HJ (1981) Carotid Doppler hemodynamics in posttraumatic intracranial hypertension. Surg Neurol 16: 459–461

195. Steiner L (1984) Treatment of arteriovenous malformations by radiosurgery. In: Wilson CB, Stein BM (eds) Intracranial arteriovenous malformations. Baltimore London, pp 295–313

196. Stephens HW Jr (1978) Electromagnetic blood flowmetry in microvascular anastomosis. In: Fein JM, Reichman OH (eds) Microvascular anastomoses for cerebral ischemia. Springer, Berlin Heidelberg New York, pp 181–194

197. Suzuki J (1979) Grading and timing of the operation on cerebral aneurysm. In: Pia HW, Langmaid J, Zierski J (eds) Cerebral aneurysm. Springer, Berlin Heidelberg New York, pp 203–208

198. Taneda M (1982) The significance of early operation in the management of ruptured intracranial aneurysm—an analysis of 251 cases hospitalized within 24 hours after subarachnoid hemorrhage. Acta Neurochir 63: 201–208

199. Tsuda Y, Kimura K, Iwata T, Haykawa T, Etanai H, Fukunaga R, Yoneda S, Abe H (1984) Improvement of cerebral blood flow and/or CO_2 reactivity after superficial artery-middle cerebral artery bypass in patients with transient ischemic attacks and watershed-zone infractions. Surg Neurol 22: 595–604

200. Uematsu S, Smith TD, Walker AE (1978) Pulsatile cerebral echo in diagnosis of brain death. J Neurosurg 48: 866–875

201. Vapalathi M, Ljunggren B, Säveland H, Hernesniemi J, Brandt L, Tapaninaho A (1984) Early aneurysm operation and outcome in two remote Scandinavian populations. J Neurosurg 60: 1160–1162

202. Volpe JJ, Perlman JM, Hill A, McMenamin JB (1982) Cerebral blood flow velocity in the human newborn: the value of its determination. Pediatrics 70: 147–152

203. Wallace JM, Nashold BS Jr, Slewka AP (1965) Hemodynamic effects of cerebral arteriovenous aneurysm. Circulation 31: 696–704

204. Weir B, Grace M, Hansen J, Rothberg Ch (1978) Time course of vasospasm in man. J Neurosurg 48: 173–178

205. Weir B (1980) The incidence and onset of vasospasm after subarachnoid hemorrhage from ruptured aneurysm. In: Wilkins RH (ed) Cerebral arterial spasm. Williams and Wilkins, Baltimore London, pp 302–305

206. White RP (1980) Overview of the pharmacology of vasospasm. In: Wilkins RH (ed), Cerebral arterial spasm. Williams and Wilkins, Baltimore London, pp 229–336

207. Wolff HP (1982) Kriterien des Hirntodes. Dtsch Ärzteblatt 79: 35–41

208. Wüllenweber R, Gött U, Wappenschmidt J (1969) Klinische, anaesthesiologische und radiologische Aspekte des Hirntodes bei traumatischen Hirnschädigungen und intrakraniellen Drucksteigerungen. In: Penin H, Käufer Ch (Hrsg) Der Hirntod. G Thieme, Stuttgart, S 23–32

209. Yamada S (1982) Arteriovenous malformations in the functional area: Surgical treatment and regional cerebral blood flow. Neurol Res 4: 283–322

210. Yamashima T, Yamamoto S (1983) Cerebral arterial pathology in experimental subarachnoid hemorrhage. J Neurosurg 58: 843–850

211. Yamashima T, Kashihara K, Ikeda K, Kubota T, Yamamoto S (1985) Three phases of cerebral arteriopathy in meningitis: Vasospasm and vasodilatation followed by organic stenosis. Neurosurgery 16: 546–553

212. Yaşargil GM (1984) Microneurosurgery, vol I. G Thieme, Stuttgart New York

213. Yoneda S, Nichimoto A, Nukada T, Kuriyama Y, Katsurada K, Abe H (1974) To-and-fro movement and external escape of carotid arterial blood in brain death cases. A Doppler ultrasonic study. Stroke 5: 707–713

214. Yoshimoto T, Uchida K, Kaneko U, Kayama T, Suzuki J (1979) An analysis of follow-up results of 1,000 intracranial saccular aneurysms with definitive surgical treatment. J Neurosurg 50: 152–157

Subject Index

ABP, arterial blood pressure   60–62
Anastomosis   78–93
   collateral flow   78, 80–85
   flow distribution   80–87
   patency   80–87
Angiography
   and TCD   1, 25, 65–69, 108–110,
    115–116
Aneurysm
   acute operation   32, 34, 40–64
   delayed operation   32, 34, 70–71
   flow pattern   72–77
   location   41
Artery, arteries
   anterior cerebral (A 1)   18, 35,
    47–51
   anterior communicating (ACoA)
    16, 35, 81–85, 96
   basilar   19–20, 24–27
   carotid, supraclinoid portion   16,
    18, 35, 47–48
   compliance   5, 118
   compression test   21–24, 78–79,
    83–85
   MCA, middle cerebral   16, 18,
    47–54, 108–110, 117–118
   PCA, posterior cerebral   18, 35,
    47–50, 87–88
   PCoA, posterior communicating
    16–18, 96
   pericallosal   45
   siphon   19, 35, 47
   vertebral   20
Autoregulation   3
   AVM and   94–96, 103, 106–107

AVM arteriovenous malformation
   94–107
   autoregulation   94–96, 103, 106–107
   CO_2-effect   96–97, 105
   embolization   94, 97–98, 103–107
   extracranial Doppler   11
   feeder   95–98, 103–106
   "normal pressure break through"
    94, 107
   steal   95–98
   velocity in feeder   95–98, 106–107

Blood flow
   CBF   1, 32, 78, 87–93
   positron emission tomography   1,
    32
Brain death   115–118
   angiography   115–116
   reverberating flow pattern   10, 60,
    62, 115–118
Bypass, see anastomosis

Carbon dioxide
   reactivity   28–29, 92–93, 96
Cerebrovascular resistance   3–4, 76,
   101–102, 117
Compression test, see Artery compression
CPP—cerebral perfusion pressure   62,
   115

Doppler
   aliasing   12, 15
   Christian   6
   continuous wave   6
   effect   6

equation 6
instrumentation 6–8, 12–15
intraoperative 1, 11, 26, 109,
  111–112
mean frequency shift 24
principle 6–7
pulsed 7
sample volume 7–9, 12
shift 6–7
spectra 8–10, 14

Extracranial-Intracranial Bypass,
  see Anastomosis

Hemorrhage
  intracerebral 52, 54
  subarachnoid 40–41
Hunt/Hess 40–41
Hypercapnia 28–29, 92–93
Hypocapnia 28–29, 92–93

ICP intracerebral pressure 11, 45, 115
Insonation angle 18–21

Jumping and TCD 30–31

Meningitis 111–114
  angiography 111
  spasm 111–114
Moya Moya 87–88
Musical Murmur 54–57

Nimodipine 40, 51–54

Occlusion
  carotid 78–93
  MCA 69
Orthostasis 29–30

Poiseulle law 3
PRF—pulse repetition frequency 7,
  12
Probe 13

Resistance
  cerebrovascular see CVR
  index 9–10, 106

SAH, subarachnoid hemmorrhage
  AVM 98–100
  location 36–37, 48–51
  source 36–39, 46, 48–51
  vasospasm, see Spasm
Skull
  bony window 14–16
  transillumination 17
Spasm
  angiography 35, 65–71
  arteries pathomorphology 33–34
  blood pressure, effect of 61–62
  cerebrovascular 32–71
  classification by TCD 59–60
  clinical significance 32, 61–64
  critical 33, 46, 59
  delayed ischemic deficit 42, 44,
    57–61
  flow reduction 46
  hemodynamic effect 33
  maximum 32, 45–63
  medical treatment 60–64
  murmur 54–57, 76–77, 100
  nimodipine 51–54, 63–64
  operation timing 32, 70–71
  side difference 46–51
  subcritical 59, 63
  surgery, effect of 32, 34, 70–71
  velocity 36
Subarachnoid Hemorrhage, see SAH

Transcranial Doppler
  comparison of intraoperative
    Doppler 26, 57, 73, 109
  examination technique 18–23
  instrumentation 12–15
  normal values 24–26
Transorbital 19–20

Vasospasm, see Spasm
Velocity
  age 27–28
  angle influence 6–7
  diastole 24
  mean 24

Velocity
 systole 24
 vector 7

Willis, Circle of 16–18

Window ultrasonic
 foramen magnum 16, 20–21
 orbital 16, 19–20
 temporal 16–19

Transcranial Doppler Sonography

Edited by **R. Aaslid**

Contents: A. Eden: The Beginnings of Doppler. – P. Grolimund: Transmission of Ultrasound Through the Temporal Bone. – R. Aaslid: The Doppler Principle Applied to Measurement of Blood Flow Velocity in Cerebral Arteries. – R. Aaslid: Transcranial Doppler Examination Techniques. – R. Aaslid, K.-F. Lindegaard: Cerebral Hemodynamics. – K.-F. Lindegaard, R. Aaslid, H. Nornes: Cerebral Arteriovenous Malformations. – J. M. Gilsbach, A. Harders: Comparison of Intraoperative and Transcranial Doppler. – R. W. Seiler, R. Aaslid: Transcranial Doppler for Evaluation of Cerebral Vasospasm. – A. Harders: Monitoring Hemodynamic Changes Related to Vasospasm in the Circle of Willis After Aneurysm Surgery. – E. B. Ringelstein: Transcranial Doppler Monitoring. – T. Lundar: Transcranial Doppler in the Study of Cerebral Perfusion During Cardiopulmonary Bypass. – Subject Index.

From the Foreword by M. P. Spencer, M. D., Director of the Institute of Applied Physiology and Medicine, Seattle, Washington, U.S.A.:
"Every few years a dissertation comes to the area of clinical application of medical technology which carries us forward as on a magic carpet into new regions of understanding and patient care. This book is such a magic carpet. It brings together, in a clear and incisive fashion, important hemodynamic principles with a simple non-invasive method of application to a part of the cerebral vasculature which has been relatively inaccessible. To the lucky and perceptive person who reads this book, a feeling of excitement and hope for progress is engendered. The diligent application of the potentials of transcranial Doppler ultrasound brings new power to our efforts in understanding the cerebral circulation and the causes, treatment and prevention of cerebrovascular disorders."

1986. 94 figures. XI, 177 pages.
ISBN 3-211-81935-5

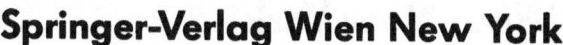

Springer-Verlag Wien New York

J. M. Gilsbach

Intraoperative
Doppler Sonography in Neurosurgery

1983. 61 figures. X, 104 pages.
ISBN 3-211-81768-9

Fully illustrated with diagrams and Doppler curve traces, "Intraoperative Doppler Sonography in Neurosurgery" demonstrates how the surgeon can improve the technique and safety of his operations with this "intravascular eye". The surgeon will no longer be dependent upon deceptive external appearances. Surgical procedures can be controlled close to the vessel allowing for an immediate decision in operative surgery.

The principles of Doppler measurement and the equipment used are discussed in great detail with emphasis on normal and pathological findings in micro-anastomoses, aneurysms, and bypass operations.

Previously unpublished information about Doppler intraoperative measurement applied to cerebrovascular operations and experimental microvascular surgery is presented in detailed case studies.

An introductory explanation is also included.

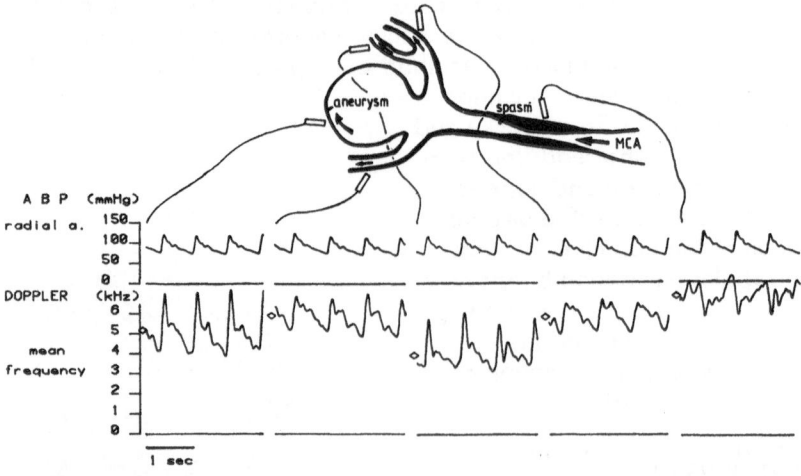

Springer-Verlag Wien New York